By The Editors of Consumer Guide®

The Dieter's Complete Guide To...
Calories, Carbohydrates, Sodium, Fats & Cholesterol

FAWCETT COLUMBINE • NEW YORK

A Fawcett Columbine Book
Published by Ballantine Books
Copyright © 1981 by Publications International, Ltd.
This book may not be reproduced or quoted in whole or in part by
mimeograph or any other printed means or for presentation on radio or
television without written permission from:
   Louis Weber, President
   Publications International, Ltd.
   3841 West Oakton Street
   Skokie, Illinois 60076
Permission is never granted for commercial purposes.

Published in the United States by Ballantine Books, a division of Random House,
Inc., New York, and in Canada by Random House of Canada, Limited, Toronto, Canada

Library of Congress Catalog Card Number: 81-80142
ISBN 0-449-90088-6

Manufactured in the United States of America

First Fawcett Columbine Edition: September 1982
First Ballantine Books Edition:
10   9   8   7   6   5   4   3

Contents

Introduction 5

Beans/Legumes 27

Beverages 28
Alcoholic Beverages • Carbonated Beverages
• Coffee and Tea • Diet and Breakfast Beverages
• Fruit and Vegetable Drinks • Fruit and Vegetable
Juices • Fruit Drink Mixes • Milk and Milk Beverages

Biscuits, Rolls, and Muffins 40
Biscuits • Cornbread • Muffins • Rolls

Breads 43
Croutons and Stuffings

Cakes and Icings 46
Cakes • Cake Mixes • Icings

Candy 51

Cereals 53
Cold, Ready-to-Eat Cereals • Hot Cereals

Cheese and Eggs 57
Natural Cheese • Processed Cheese and Spreads
• Eggs

Condiments and Baking Products 61

Cookies 65
Cookie Doughs • Cookie Mixes

Crackers 70
Toasts

Cream and Yogurt 73

Fast Foods 75

Fats, Oils, and Shortenings 79
Butter • Margarine

4 CONTENTS

Fish and Seafood 81

Flours, Meals, and Grains 87
    Flours • Rice and Rice Dishes

Fruits 91

Gelatins and Puddings 102

Gravies and Other Sauces 105

Ice Cream 107
    Frozen Desserts • Ice Cream • Ice Milk

Jellies and Jams 110

Meals and Entrees 111
    Entrees • Frozen Meals • Pizzas

Meats 119
    Beef • Lamb • Pork • Veal

Nuts and Seeds 128

Pancakes and Waffles 130

Pasta and Pasta Dishes 131

Pies and Pastries 135

Poultry 142
    Chicken • Turkey

Salad Dressings 146

Sausages and Luncheon Meats 151

Snack Foods 158

Soups and Broths 162

Sugars, Sweeteners, and Toppings 172
    Dessert Toppings • Sugars and Sweeteners • Syrups

Vegetables 176
    Vegetable Dishes and Combinations

Introduction

For better or worse, we are what we eat. New reports from scientists demonstrating ever more connections between the food we eat and the state of our health seem to appear daily. A host of diseases may be affected by food intake, including high blood pressure, diabetes, coronary artery disease, and obesity. Learning to eat properly is the important first step toward attaining your proper weight and a healthy lifestyle. Stop and think about what you eat. Then take charge of what and how much goes on your plate and palate. Those excess calories could wind up on your hips. Shop wisely and stock your pantry with nutritious, satisfying foods. You'll find it doesn't take long to point your diet in the right direction.

NUTRIENTS WE NEED

To help you make informed food choices, let's begin with a brief guide to nutrition. What foods are necessary for good health, whether you want to lose, gain, or simply maintain your weight?

We've come a long way toward identifying substances we require and their necessary amounts. Research has resulted in recommended daily allowances (RDAs) of vitamins, minerals, and protein needed to maintain health for infants, children, and adults. While these RDAs are useful, much more information is still needed to translate body requirements into beneficial eating habits.

To help us choose the necessary foods, nutritionists have divided foods into several groups. Some speak of seven food groups, others mention four. We believe the most useful system for American adults has five food groups. The accompanying chart lists these, plus serving size, dietary contribution, and recommended number of servings per day. The first four food groups—fruits and vegetables; bread and cereal; milk and cheese; and meat, fish, poultry, and beans—provide essential nutrients. To remain healthy, everyone should eat the prescribed number of daily servings of each of those groups. This means

THE FIVE FOOD GROUPS

Food Groups	Serving Sizes	Major Dietary Contribution	Recommended Servings Per Day
1 Fruits Vegetables	½ cup, 1 orange, ½ grapefruit, 1 wedge lettuce 1 bowl salad	Vitamins C and A Fiber	4 (including 1 good Vitamin C source)
2 Bread Cereal	1 slice bread 1 oz. cold cereal ½-¾ cup cooked cereal, cornmeal, grits, macaroni, rice, spaghetti	B Vitamins Iron Protein Fiber	4 (including some whole grain bread or cereal)
3 Milk Cheese	1 cup milk or yogurt 1⅓ oz. cheddar or Swiss cheese	Calcium Vitamins A, B_6 and B_{12}, D Riboflavin	Children under 9 and adults: 2 Children 9-12 and pregnant women: 3 Teens and nursing mothers: 4
4 Meat Fish Poultry Beans	2-3 oz. lean, boneless meat 2 eggs 1-1½ cups cooked beans 4-6 Tbsp. peanut butter	Protein Phosphorus Vitamins B_6, B_{12} and others Iron	2 (varying the choices among these foods)
5 Fats Sweets Alcohol	Butter, margarine, mayonnaise, candy, jams, syrups, soft drinks, liquor. Also refined but unenriched breads & pastry	Mainly calories Vitamin E and essential fatty acids from vegetable oils	None (variable)

Source: U.S. Department of Agriculture, *Home and Garden Bulletin Number 228.*

that whether you are trying to lose or gain weight, you should have four servings of each of the first two groups and two servings of groups three and four.

The fifth group in the chart includes fats, sweets, and alcoholic beverages. These are foods which contribute very little nutritionally, aside from substantial calories (see below). This food group is not mentioned in the old four-food system we all learned in school, but it is especially important to the millions of American adults who want to lose or keep down their weight. Creating a sensible diet means seriously cutting back, or even temporarily eliminating, these "foods." Dieters who are not told this crucial fact are being deluded.

Using these food groups is an easy way to decide what and how to eat. Certainly, everyone can recognize the nutritional values and roles of simple foods, such as a piece of fruit or chicken. However, most food is not eaten in a pure and simple state. It is prepared first, be it in the kitchen at home, at a restaurant, or at a cannery or packager. The fruit becomes a pie; the chicken is fried. While the slice of fruit pie you eat may provide you with a serving of Group 1 fruit, you are also getting unenriched pastry from Group 5. Likewise, the fried chicken provides a serving of meat (Group 4), but it also contains additional fat (Group 5).

While planning your diet around getting the essential nutrients, you also may want to avoid or limit your consumption of certain food factors, such as calories, carbohydrates, sodium, fat, and cholesterol. The following discussion of these food factors may be a useful guide.

CALORIES

Calories are not actually contained in food. Rather, they are a measure of the energy we can obtain from food. Actually, calories are a byproduct of the chemical changes which our bodies produce on the food we eat. Calories or energy are derived from fat, carbohydrates (including sugar), and protein. For each gram (1/28 ounce) of fat we eat, we produce about nine calories of energy. From each gram of carbohydrate or protein, we can derive approximately 4 calories of energy.

From these calorie sources, we obtain the energy needed to maintain body heat, digest food, and carry on our activities. The colder our surroundings or the more active we are, the more calories we use. If we use up more calories than we can obtain from the food we eat, we get more energy by metabolizing our body fat. This is how we lose weight. On the other hand, if the food we eat provides us with more calories than we can use at the moment, our body wisely stores those calories in the form of fat. We can draw on this energy store between meals and overnight.

When our intake of energy sources—fat, carbohydrate, and protein—exceeds our energy needs too greatly, we get a noticeable accumulation of body fat. The only way to get rid of that excess fat is to reverse the process. If you eat less of the energy sources than can fulfill your energy needs (or spend more energy on exercise), then you use up body fat.

CARBOHYDRATE

Most foods contain carbohydrate, the name for a broad group of compounds which includes starches and sugars. The most common sugar is table sugar or sucrose, the chemical combination of glucose and fructose. (Glucose is the sugar referred to in the term blood sugar, and is the body's major source of energy.) The body easily and rapidly interconverts glucose and fructose, both of which provide four calories of energy for each gram of sugar metabolized by the body. Some starch is metabolized to sugar; other starch is not metabolized in our bodies and is termed fiber. Fiber passes through the digestive tract and into the feces intact. Most of the starch in breads and pastry made with refined flour is metabolized; it provides a high calorie load and negligible fiber. In contrast, much of the starch present in fruits and vegetables is indigestible fiber, which accounts for their modest calorie contribution to the diet and their reputation for adding bulk to the digestive tract.

Everyone needs carbohydrate every day. And the latest federal government recommendations call for greater consumption of "complex carbohydrates"—the natural sugars and starches found in fruits, vegetables and whole grains. This recommendation does *not* mean we should eat more pie and cake.

Currently our American diet is saturated with processed sugar, a nutritionally empty food from Group 5. Food manufacturers claim that the addition of sugar to processed foods makes them more palatable. Hence, sugar is added to many foods, even those that don't taste sweet.

It's important to realize that sugar goes by many names. Learn to recognize them so you can identify even its "hidden" presence on the labels required for commercially prepared foods. Refined sugar may be listed as sucrose, dextrose, fructose, invert sugar, sorbitol, xylose, corn syrup, corn sweetener, natural sweetener, or lactose (milk sugar).

Recently, "natural sweeteners" have been promoted as nutritionally more acceptable. These usually refer to molasses, honey, and fructose, though all sugar comes from natural sources. As we see it, honey offers no basic advantage over refined corn syrup or sugar obtained from beets or sugar cane. Molasses, too, is primarily a calorie source; however, its high mineral content may be beneficial to some individuals. Far from being especially natural, fructose that is obtained by separation from glucose or sucrose is one of the most processed sugars available!

SODIUM

Sodium is a dietary nutrient present in most foods and especially in table salt (sodium chloride). One level teaspoon of salt contains about 2,000 milligrams of sodium. Only recently has medical science come to realize the dietary importance of this mineral.

As with many things, we consume far more sodium than we need; and scientists now say that this overuse may be a major cause of hypertension—high bood pressure. The U.S. Senate Select Committee on Nutrition has recommended reducing salt consumption to a daily goal of 3 grams, or about 1,200 milligrams of sodium. The standard American diet contains 2,300 to 6,900 milligrams of sodium per day. While it is not certain that excess sodium causes hypertension, it has no beneficial effect either. To be safe, extra sodium should be avoided.

Sodium is present in virtually all natural and manmade foods. It is present in drinking water and is added to softened water. Fresh meat, fish, poultry, and eggs contain substantial amounts of sodium. However, only small amounts of sodium are present in most fresh fruits, vegetables, and grains. Frequently, much sodium is added to commercially processed food; hence canned or frozen fruits and vegetables, as well as processed grains, can have high sodium contents. Frozen fish, which is frequently washed in brine (salt water), may have a very high sodium content.

Most recipes call for salt; so even if you can't taste it, the cook or chef has no doubt added sodium to virtually any dish. Importantly, many Americans salt their food heavily at the table. By limiting the addition of salt in cooking and simply removing the table salt shaker, many persons could cut in half their sodium intake. For stringent, sodium-restricted diets, your doctor will usually insist you avoid any processed foods with a high sodium content, cook your own food without salt, and take the salt shaker off the table. If your water supply is salty (check with your local board of health), you may even need to use mineral-free distilled water.

FATS

Fat, which serves up more than twice as many calories as do protein or carbohydrates, is the most fattening food there is. While some fat in the diet is essential to nutrition, "getting the fat out" is still the most surefire method for eliminating unwanted calories.

In its *Dietary Goals for the U.S.*, the Senate Select Committee on Nutrition urged a cutback in fat intake so that it supplies 30 percent, rather than 40 percent, of your energy needs.

Pure fat gives you nine calories per gram while so-called pure carbohydrate and protein provide only four calories. Or, to translate these numbers into pounds, a pound of oil or shortening supplies about 4,000 calories, while a pound of pure carbohydrate or protein gives you 1,800. Actually no food is pure, unadulterated carbohydrate or protein. And some foods we usually think of as protein, such as meat, provide more fat calories than protein calories. However, some protein foods contain very little fat. Two examples are shellfish such as abalone (about 83 percent solids) and dried egg whites (80 percent protein).

Remember, though, that fat is fat; regardless of type, it is high in calories. Margarine (vegetable fat) and butter (animal fat) both supply 100 calories per tablespoon. The emphasis on vegetable fat for diet purposes has nothing to do with cutting calories or losing weight but rather with what seems to be the cholesterol-lowering ability of polyunsaturated vegetable fats when used in place of animal fats. Studies have shown that it's possible to help lower a person's cholesterol level by substituting polyunsaturated fats for saturated animal fats.

While the calories are the same, there are basic differences in the chemical structure of different types of fats. Fats are divided into three types: saturated, monounsaturated and polyunsaturated. Saturated fats are generally believed to be the villains that help raise cholesterol levels. Saturated fats are usually solid at room temperature; they include all forms of animal fat—including butter; the fat in milk, cream, and cheese; and the fat encasing and marbling meats. Poultry fats and fish oils are softer than meat fat and less saturated, but just as fattening. A few vegetable fats are also highly saturated: for example, coconut oil, cocoa butter and hydrogenated vegetable fats (solid shortenings).

Olive oil and peanut oil are high in monounsaturated fats.

Monounsaturated fats are neutral in effect, neither raising nor lowering your cholesterol level. Polyunsaturated fats, on the other hand, have been demonstrated to help lower cholesterol levels. These are usually liquid oils of vegetable origin and include safflower, corn, cottonseed, sesame, and sunflower seed oils. Safflower oil is the highest in polyunsaturates.

As we have said, the number of calories does not vary with the type of fat. A low fat diet seeks to eliminate excess calories by reducing the amount of fat consumed. And a low-saturated-fat diet may help lower the cholesterol level.

CHOLESTEROL

Cholesterol itself is a normal constituent of the cells of human and animal life. Thus, foods of animal and fish origin contain cholesterol in varying amounts. Foods of plant origin—such as fruits, vegetables, grains, legumes, nuts, and even highly saturated coconut oil—do *not* contain cholesterol. While cholesterol and saturated fat are often found together in animal foods, their quantities are not dependent on one another. Thus, one large egg contains approximately 2 grams of saturated fat and 250 milligrams of cholesterol, while one cup of whole milk contains approximately 5 grams of saturated fat and only 34 milligrams of cholesterol.

Thus, because cholesterol and saturated fat are found together, a cholesterol-lowering diet is one in which the total amount of fats—particularly saturated fats—is decreased, while the proportion of polyunsaturated fat intake is increased. At the same time, foods containing substantial amounts of cholesterol are used in moderation. Evidence of the role of cholesterol-lowering diets in preventing heart disease is mounting and, therefore, it is prudent to use fats or oils that are primarily polyunsaturated—particularly safflower and corn oils and margarines made from them.

At this point, it would be advantageous to clear up what seems to be a rather widespread misconception concerning the amount of cholesterol found in shellfish. Except for shrimp, the commonly eaten "shellfish" (oysters, clams, scallops, lobster, and crab) are not totally prohibited for those on cholesterol-restricted diets. These shellfish can be used interchangeably with allowable types of meat. Shrimp is moderately high in cholesterol—compared to organ meats, such as liver, kidney, heart, and brains, which are very high in cholesterol content—and its consumption should be limited.

NUTRITION LABELING

Learn to read the fine print on package labels. If you're a bargain hunter by instinct, you're already experienced in comparing packages and prices, weights and measures. You use that information to identify the best buy for the money. You'll find it's easy to transfer those same skills to become a calorie-comparison shopper. Just as you look for the most value for your money, you will also look for the most nutrition for your calories. This approach can save you literally hundreds of thousands of calories a year.

Now that many foods are labeled with nutritional data, it's easier to make calorie and fat comparisons among competing grocery items. By law, any product that makes a nutrition claim ("low calorie," "lower in fat," "higher in protein," "high in vitamin C," for example) must also include complete nutritional information in accordance with a legally defined format. "Low calorie" means that a food provides 40 calories or fewer per serving and that each gram of food (1/28 ounce) gives 0.4 calories or fewer. "Reduced calorie" means that the labeled food has at least one third fewer the number of calories found in the regular item. For example, jam providing 29 calories per tablespoon is a "reduced calorie" product compared to regular jam with 55 calories per tablespoon.

Look behind the words "dietetic," "lower in fat," "lower in saturated fat," "no butterfat," "nondairy," "part skim" and "sugar-free." Check the nutrition label, and find out exactly what these catch words mean. These special products usually cost more, so find out what you are paying for. "Dietetic" does not necessarily mean low in calories; it may mean salt-free or sweetened with sorbitol. The latter may help diabetics, but the number of calories is the same as for regular sugar. Some dietetic foods are just as fattening as nondietetic foods. Even if a particular brand of product is "lower in fat," it still could be relatively high in calories. Some dairy product substitutes are lower in saturated fat or labeled "no butterfat" but contain vegetable oil instead and are just as fattening as others. For example, specially formulated mayonnaise substitutes may lack eggs and saturated fat, but can be just as rich in calories. Or, a truly low fat product may be high in calories because of added sugar. On the other hand, sugar-free products can be calorie-rich because of added fat. If you want to lose weight, the real "bottom line" to watch is the calorie count; compare it with that of a competing product.

Beware of Unlabeled Products. If the manufacturer makes no nutritional claims for its product, then nutritional labeling is voluntary. Many food manufacturers include nutritional data, even though not required. A food company willing to disclose complete information about its product may inspire more confidence than one that doesn't. Thus, a shopper is inclined to believe that the nutritionally labeled food offers more nutrition than the product of the competitor who isn't willing to disclose the information. However, until all foods are labeled, we just won't know.

Especially in diet shops and health food stores, unlabeled products represent a potential trap. You may expect all products to be "dietetic" or "natural," but this is not always true. Don't trust the verbal claims of clerks or hand-lettered signs stating the veal sausage, beef bologna, or artichoke spaghetti is low-calorie, unless you are shown actual product labeling. If the particular product being sold is substantially lower in calories, the store manager can support the claim with a printed packing crate label or other official information from the manufacturer. Sometimes the deception is unintentional; the clerk or counterperson may assume that the product is low in calories because of how it is sold.

To help you through the confusing array of labeled and unlabeled products, we present a brief guide to dairy products, bread, fruits and vegetables, meat and poultry, and other foods.

DAIRY PRODUCTS

Once upon a time there were only three kinds of milk, and they all came in the same bottle: the kind at the top, the kind at the bottom, and the kind you got when you shook up the bottle.

Today the dairy section is more like an enchanted dairyland of eggs, egg substitutes, creams, coffee lighteners, nondairy substitutes, whipped toppings, yogurts, ice milk, and dietetic frozen desserts. There are imported cheeses, imitation cheeses, processed cheeses, and so-called cheese foods. In addition, there are many ways to buy milk: skimmed, low fat, dried, evaporated, condensed, sweetened, cultured, malted, flavored, with 2 percent butterfat, with 1 percent butterfat, with added Vitamins A and D and nonfat dry milk solids.

This bewildering assortment of dairy and nondairy alternatives results from needs of various groups of consumers to cut down on fat, saturated fat, cholesterol, and/or calories. To meet these requirements, a variety of products with cross-purposes have been created. Unless you have a clear idea of what you wish to avoid, it's easy to pay a premium price for an alternative you don't want. For example, you may think an item is low in calories, only to discover after months of use that it's even more fattening than the product you had used previously. You may select a cholesterol-free nondairy imitation product, not knowing that it's full of cholesterol-raising saturated fat. Luckily, much of the information you really need to know is on the label—even if in small print.

Milk. We are told that we never outgrow our need for milk. But since most of the important nutrients in milk are available elsewhere, or in other dairy products, that statement is open to debate. Nevertheless, milk is a significant source of low-cost protein and calcium. If you choose a defatted or low fat version, milk can also be a low fat, low calorie beverage. Skim milk has about half the calories of whole milk, yet it contains just as much protein and calcium. Only fat (and fat calories) are removed.

About Powdered Milk. The calorie, fat, and cholesterol data for reconstituted (following package directions) nonfat dry milks are approximately the same as that for fresh skim milk. There are two types of nonfat dry milk available. Instant nonfat dry milk, sold in supermarkets, is heat-treated so that it dissolves easily in cold water. Noninstant is harder to find, but some people find its flavor superior, much closer to that of fresh milk. (Noninstant or nonheat-treated dry milk is usually sold in health food stores.) It takes less of the noninstant powder to make one cup of milk— only ¼ cup compared with ⅓ cup of the dry instant milk. When reconstituted according to package directions, both milks have approximately the same nutritional content.

How to Lighten Your Coffee. To our way of thinking, the most nutritious, least fattening way to lighten coffee (or tea) is with low fat fresh milk. A tablespoon provides only about 6 calories and ½ milligram of cholesterol.

Yogurt. Yogurt, plain and simple, is fermented milk that has no more nutritional value than the milk it was made from. It is fermented by the addition of "friendly" bacteria. These bacteria digest the milk, thickening it somewhat and changing its taste from fresh to slightly tart or sour. With the action of these friendly bacteria on the milk, yogurt becomes easier for the human body to digest. Since yogurt is usually (but not always) made from low fat milk, it would be an excellent snack if people simply ate it plain. However, most of the yogurt sold in this country has been calorie-inflated with sugar-laden fruit preserves. The flavorings and sweeteners can double the calorie count.

Eggs and Egg Substitutes. At only 82 calories apiece and less than 12 percent fat, eggs are certainly one of the leanest, least fattening main courses a calorie-counter could choose—and one of the most controversial! The problem, of course, is the cholesterol. The fact that the yolk of an egg contains about 250 milligrams of cholesterol has prompted the American Heart Association to suggest limiting egg yolk consumption to three a week. (The white of the egg does not contain cholesterol.) The egg industry has countered with promotional campaigns assuring shoppers that eggs are a valuable, nutritious food, and that there's no proof that curtailing egg consumption will save you from developing heart disease. There are eminent scientists on either side of the fence. If you *are* limiting the amount of cholesterol in your diet, you should probably follow the recommendations for limiting the number of eggs you eat.

For the cholesterol-conscious or egg-yolk-allergic, egg substitutes are a boon that allows the enjoyment of scrambled "eggs" for breakfast or an omelet for lunch or supper. These products are formulated to look, taste, and cook like eggs, so they can be used in place of eggs in many recipes where whole eggs are used as a binder. However, you should check the calorie count of the egg substitute you select. Convenient as they are for cholesterol-watchers, some brands of egg substitute are no bargain for calorie-counters. Some egg substitutes actually contain more fat and calories than an equivalent amount of eggs. All egg substitutes are nutritionally labeled, so check the calorie and fat information and pick the brand with the least calories. (Keep in mind that one large fresh egg has about 80 calories, 6 grams of protein, and 6 grams of fat.)

Shopping for Cheeses. For the serious fat-fighter, most cheeses are a caloric extravagance to be used sparingly, more as a seasoning than a food. An important exception is, of course, cottage cheese, which well deserves its reputation as the fat-fighter's friend. Also, mozzarella and ricotta, made partly from skim milk, are lower in fat and calories. Feta cheese and Neufchatel cheese are somewhat lower in fat and calorie content, too.

Don't be turned away by the word "imitation" on cheeses. There is a real need for cheeses with a reduced fat and calorie content, and a number of brands are available in different sections of the country. They are labeled "imitation cheese" only because they contain less butterfat than required by the official standards for cheeses. In other words, if you make a Cheddar that's identical to other Cheddars in every way except that it contains less fat, the cheese must be labeled "imitation"—even though it is nutritionally superior (having less fat and more protein) to the traditional Cheddar.

If you are trying to save calories, beware of the reduced-butterfat cheeses to which polyunsaturated fats have been added. Although these might be useful to a cholesterol-watcher without a weight problem, a person who is trying to lose weight by eating less fat will not save anything by buying them. These cheeses are usually well labeled. If weight is your primary concern, always watch for fat and calorie data.

Because salt (sodium chloride) is used in its manufacturing, cheese tends to have a higher sodium content than many foods. Fat and calorie contents are not accurate guides to sodium content in cheese. In a cheese labeled "low-sodium," a salt substitute (usually potassium chloride) has been used in the manufacturing process as partial replacement for sodium chloride.

BREAD

Generations of dieters have shunned bread needlessly, when the real calorie culprit was what they spread on it! With bread goes butter or margarine—at 100 calories per level tablespoon—or peanut butter at 95 calories and jelly at 55 calories.

To avoid unnecessary calories, eat bread without the spread. Instead use bread and bread products in sandwiches filled with high-protein lean meat, poultry, or seafood. Bread is also a good meat stretcher: top it with slices of lean roast and low fat gravy for a hot sandwich main course.

There are differences in breads, and the would-be waistline-watcher should choose the types made with enriched and/or whole grain flour and minimal or no added fat and sugar. Check the label for nutrition information. And remember, calories and fat content vary with the size of the loaf or the thickness of the slice.

FRUITS AND VEGETABLES

Fruits and vegetables are low in calories and fat and high in vitamins. They help you meet your daily vitamin requirements—with fewer calories and less fat than any other type of food.

Fruits and vegetables—in and of themselves—are filling. Fifty calories' worth of steak or cake is a small piece which barely makes a dent in your appetite. But there's not much room for overeating after you've put away a large 50-calorie bowl of salad greens. And fruits and vegetables take time to eat. The 50-calorie salad takes much longer to chew than a 50-calorie mouthful of meat or dessert.

Fresh fruits and vegetables are also the most significant source of food fiber, an important element that's been refined out of America's over-processed food products. Fiber—or roughage—is the non-nutritive, indigestible residue found in most fruits and vegetables, seeds, nuts, and whole grains. Since fiber is neither vitamin, mineral, or protein, food makers seldom bother to list fiber content on their labels. The true fiber content of most foods will be known only as more attention is given to this important substance.

One thing fiber does is help to fill you up. What better way to reduce the likelihood of overeating? For example, eating a big salad along with your steak can mean you will be satisfied with a smaller steak. But there's more. Fiber tends to speed up the passage of foods through your digestive system, acting as a cleanser. Recent research points to the value of fiber in the diet of some primitive societies where life expectancy is long and many of our modern diseases are unknown. These people's natural diets consist of fruits, vegetables, nuts, and grains in abundance, but little meats and sweets.

MEATS

Meat is important for providing protein, but much of it is also high in fat. You can cut calories simply by cutting down on the quantity of meat served. Two ways to do this are eliminating meat from some meals and serving smaller portions. Smaller portions go unnoticed when you have a wider choice of other filling foods as side dishes: soups, salads, a variety of interesting vegetables, potatoes, pasta or rice prepared in nonfattening ways, breads, and fresh-fruit desserts. Even a seven-course banquet can add up to fewer calories if a variety of foods takes the place of second and third helpings of meat. But even if you don't eat less meat, you can slash calories by choosing meat for its nutritional quality (low fat content).

Saving Calories with the Right Cuts. Selecting the right cut of any meat can save you more calories than simply avoiding certain types of meat. It's an oversimplification to say that beef is more fattening than veal or that ham is more fattening than lamb. Although veal is generally leaner than beef, some cuts of veal are fatter and higher in calories than some cuts of beef. And some cuts of pork are leaner than some cuts of beef or lamb. If you know the best cuts of each meat to choose, and the best ways to cook them, you can broaden your meat choices. Here are a few simple guidelines:

1. Younger is leaner than older. Animals, like people, tend to add fat as they age. For that reason, a veal or lamb rib chop is less fattening than a beef or pork rib chop, because it comes

from young animals. Young frying chickens are markedly less fattening than older stewing chickens.

2. The leaner and less fattening tender cuts of meat come from the rear—from the leg. This applies to meat animals—beef, veal, lamb, pork, ham—not poultry. A leg cut of beef is called beef round. In veal, it is called veal round. In lamb, it's a leg steak or leg chop, and in pork it's called a fresh ham slice. (The word ham refers to a leg cut of pork, not whether it's cured or smoked. A *cured* ham slice would be called a smoked ham slice.)

3. The most fattening tender cuts come from the middle—from the rib. Rib steaks and rib chops of all meat animals generally have the highest fat content and give you the most calories.

4. The less fattening, less tender cuts come from the front end—from the arm and shoulder. Of these, the cuts from the arm or foreshank are less fattening than the shoulder. Beef cuts from this area are known as chuck. In pork, it's sometimes called picnic.

5. The most fattening, least tender cuts come from the underbelly. This includes beef brisket and short plate, from which corned beef and pastrami are usually made. Also laden with fat are breast of veal and lamb, pork spareribs, and bacon. One outstanding exception from the underbelly of beef is flank steak, an exceedingly lean and tender steak. It's virtually free of visible fat. It's also the leanest and least fattening of all beef cuts—a real find for beef lovers who are fat-fighters.

How to Buy Hamburger. According to federal law, hamburger may contain up to 30 percent fat. State and local laws sometimes impose a 25-percent fat limit, but that still represents a lot of fat. And unfortunately, the ground meat you take home may even exceed the legal limit; stores are occasionally cited for such infractions. Many grocery chains offer premium-priced lean or diet hamburger; but the fat content is usually at least 10 percent, sometimes 15 percent or more.

The safest way for a fat-fighter to buy hamburger is to select a lean bottom round or chuck roast, have it trimmed of fat and ground to order. This special order hamburger will be less fattening and usually no more expensive than the ready-ground premium-lean meats. Bottom round is leaner and more expensive than chuck, but the calorie savings are worth it.

What really counts most is your own eyeball inspection of the meat you choose for grinding. You may get lucky and find a bargain-priced chuck that's actually leaner than a bottom round steak. Because all packaged roasts contain some fat, look for a roast where the fat can be trimmed—situated around the meat, not marbled throughout.

POULTRY

Compared with most meats, all chicken is relatively low in fat and calories, but your best bet is young frying chickens. (You can use a frying chicken in place of any other chicken, if you just reduce the cooking time for this tender bird.) Don't let the word fryer mislead you; you don't need to fry it! If you are cutting calories, frying is the one thing you don't want to do with it! The word fryer simply refers to age. Frying chickens are young and tender enough to quick-cook in high heat. They are also ideal for broiling or cooking on the grill.

The breast is the leanest meat on the chicken, and so the lowest in calories, fat, and waste. All in all, chicken meat is so low in calories and fat that you can enjoy the other parts as well. Listed in order of fat content—from least fat to most fat—poultry parts rank as follows: (1)breast, (2)drumstick, (3)thigh, (4)wing, (5)neck, and (6)back. You can shave calories from all chicken pieces by discarding the skin to which much of the fat is attached.

Younger turkeys have proportionally less fat and fewer calories per pound of meat than older turkeys. Contrary to popular opinion, young birds have the same proportion of meat-to-bone as older birds. In other words, you're not getting more meat and less bone with older birds; what you are getting is more fat. Unfortunately, lean younger turkeys cost more per pound than older ones.

Here's where you can save cash as well as calories and cholesterol. Do not waste money and calories on self-basting turkeys which have been artificially pumped full of oil and additives. Despite the tempting claims of butter on self-basters' labels, the fat generally is not butter. Also, those who have been cautioned to watch sodium intake should be wary of basted birds because the baste usually is high in sodium.

FISH AND SEAFOOD

Compared with most meats, virtually all seafood is low in fat and calories. Even supposedly fatty fish such as salmon, bluefish, and mackerel seem like diet fare by comparison with most meats. Mackerel, for example, is only 12 percent fat. The fat content of cod is so low that it's measured in fractions of a percent. So a fat-fighter can enjoy any seafood that's available, as long as the cooking method doesn't inflate the calorie count excessively.

For those on cholesterol- or sodium-restricted diets, however, there are some special considerations. Shrimp is moderately high in cholesterol; its use should be limited if you are on a low-cholesterol diet. All shellfish are relatively high in sodium and are, therefore, usually not recommended for low-sodium diets. Also, during the freezing process, fish frequently are washed in brine, thus pushing the sodium content to an unacceptably high level for low-sodium diets. We suggest that you always use fresh fish if you are restricting your sodium intake.

PASTA, RICE, AND POTATOES

Despite the fattening reputation of potatoes, rice, spaghetti, macaroni, noodles, and other pasta products, these foods are virtually fat free. It is the rich sauces or other fatty ingredients that add most of the calories to pasta dishes. If you combine potatoes, rice, or pasta with low fat, low calorie ingredients or with homemade, fat-skimmed sauces, you can enjoy these foods often *and* watch your weight.

Most spaghetti-type products, despite differences in shape—shells, strips, tubes, wheels or whatever—"weigh in" at about 105 calories per ounce of dry pasta. If you cook spaghetti products longer than the recommended time—14 to 20 minutes to the tender stage, rather than 8 to 10 minutes to the firm stage or *al dente*—they will absorb more water and swell to a larger size. For that reason, one cupful of tender-cooked spaghetti is lower in calories than a cupful cooked *al dente*—155 calories instead of 215 calories.

FROZEN DESSERTS

There's a confusing array of frozen desserts available to dieters. What to choose depends on what you want to avoid: Is it calories, cholesterol, fat, or sugar? Don't be misled—read the nutrition labels carefully. A frozen dessert that's almost fat-free may be high in sugar and nearly as fattening as your favorite ice cream. A "dietetic" or low-sugar sweet may be rich with butterfat.

If you want to avoid cholesterol, choose ices, ice milk, low fat frozen yogurt, or sherbet. Avoid ice cream, and especially avoid frozen custard, which is made with egg yolks.

If you want to avoid fat, choose ices, low fat frozen yogurt, low fat ice milk or sherbet. Avoid ice cream, especially the more expensive high-fat brands.

If you want to avoid sugar, choose sugar-free dietetic ice milk or ice cream. Avoid ices, sherbets, frozen yogurt and regular ice cream or ice milk.

If you want to avoid calories, choose low fat ice milk—the lower the fat content, the better.

LOW CALORIE DIET FOODS

Look for calorie-saving products on the diet shelf in categories such as those listed below.

A. Canned fruits packed in water or juice instead of syrup provide less than half the calories of syrup-packed fruits.

B. Low calorie, low fat diet salad dressings formulated with less or no oil.

C. Diet sodas and soft drinks made without sugar.

D. Regular or instant sugar-free iced tea mix made without sugar. Better yet, brew your own.

E. Sugar-free, low fat hot cocoa and milkshake mixes made with nonfat milk powder.

F. Sugar-free gelatin and pudding mixes.

G. Calorie-reduced cake mixes with labels indicating the product is low in fat and sweetened with a small amount of fructose, rather than those sweetened with sorbitol sweetener (for diabetics).

H. Low calorie pancake mixes and sugar-free pancake syrups.

I. Diet cheeses which are specially formulated to be low fat and clearly labeled with pertinent information.

J. Low-sugar and sugar-free jams, jellies, preserves, and spreads.

K. Diet margarines, which usually contain half the calories of regular margarines or butter.

L. Low calorie frozen desserts, including ice milks and frozen yogurt. Look for a brand with less than 2 percent fat and a labeled calorie count under 100 per half-cup serving.

IN HEALTH FOOD STORES

If you wish to avoid excess calories, fat, and sugar, keep in mind that even natural foods can be fattening, and that "natural" is sometimes used indiscriminately or attributed with miracle powers. Some "health foods" contain more fat and sweetening ingredients than their supermarket counterparts. Some granola-type cereals, for example, are sprinkled with oil and honey and contain nearly 500 calories a cupful compared with 110 calories in corn flakes or 90 in Kellogg's Special K breakfast cereal. While granola is nutritious, its high calorie and fat content would make it more suitable for youngsters, athletes or other highly active people not engaged in fighting excess weight.

At health food stores, as everywhere, informed buying is important. Despite their higher price, some health food products are real calorie bargains. Look for the following:

A. Dried fruits: Those prepared without sugar are great for making low calorie sweets and treats. Health food stores generally offer a wider variety of dried fruits. People following low-sodium diets may find dried fruit without the sodium sulfite preservative.

B. Natural fruit juices and concentrates: Health food stores generally offer varieties made without sugar or other sweeteners that may not be available at retail stores.

C. Soy flour is higher in protein than wheat flour. Adding low fat protein to your menus in this form allows you to meet your protein requirement with less meat, while cutting down on cholesterol and saturated fat.

D. Whole-grain flour and cereals: Whole-wheat flour, stone-ground corn meal, brown rice, natural oatmeal, grits, and other minimally processed grain products are richer in many nutrients (and fiber) than the refined products. Be wary, however, of mixes. The mixes generally contain added oil, sugar, and salt—more than you would need to use if you were to prepare the item from scratch.

E. Fructose or "fruit sugar": For the same quantity and calories, fructose is 1½ times sweeter than table sugar (sucrose) when used to sweeten fruits and other acid foods. This makes it a better choice than ordinary table sugar, if you actually use less. Like sucrose, fructose is pure calories and should be used sparingly. It is much more expensive than sucrose. Raw sugar and turbinado sugar are no sweeter than table sugar; and their miniscule amounts of nutritional substances do not make up for their high calories.

IN RESTAURANTS

An ever-increasing share of America's food dollars is spent in restaurants rather than in supermarkets and food stores. This has been attributed to increases in the numbers of singles, working wives, childless couples, and business travelers.

There are two types of restaurant dining to consider: the routine refueling stops—breakfast on the road or lunch at the office—and the kind you do for the fun of it—dining with friends, trying new restaurants, sampling local specialties, celebrating special occasions.

Of the two, the routine refueling stops represent the greater threat of excess fat and calories. For example, many fast-food places specialize in the quick-cooking, deep-fried fare that is high in fat and calories. However, the multi-course, gourmet-food dinner can also be a high-calorie trap.

Following are some suggestions for low calorie selections to seek out and some calorific disasters to avoid. If you give it a little thought, dining out can still be both pleasurable and healthful.

Breakfast. GOOD CHOICES: fresh fruit, cereal with milk (especially a high-protein cereal), poached or soft-cooked egg (unless you're cholesterol-watching). The least fattening breakfast meats available in commercial eating places are Canadian bacon and ham. Order unbuttered toast or English muffins—or, better yet, bagels, which are higher in protein. AVOID: fried eggs (they're almost always fried in too much fat), pancakes or French toast with syrup, bacon, sausage, Danish pastries, prebuttered toast, bread or rolls, and jams or jellies.

Quick Lunches. GOOD CHOICES: chef's salad with dressing on the side (add only a tablespoon or request the low-calorie dressing), cottage cheese with fresh fruit (avoid canned or sweetened fruit), sandwiches made with lean meats like turkey, roast beef, chicken, or boiled ham. Ask for a pickle on the side and lettuce and tomato in the sandwich. AVOID: hot dogs, hamburgers, French fries, and anything else deep-fat fried. Avoid sausages and lunchmeats; those available at the average lunch counter are likely to be high in fat and calories. Avoid salad fillings made with mayonnaise.

Dinner. GOOD CHOICES: broiled seafood or chicken, roast turkey, veal steak or chops, lean roast beef, liver (if you are not restricting cholesterol), small tenderloin steak, flank steak, London broil. Look for places with good salad bars. Then supplement your entree with salad greens, tomatoes, carrots, celery, mushrooms, and other fresh vegetables. AVOID: breaded and deep-fat fried entrees and side dishes, most casserole-style combination dishes made with sauces or cheeses, steak and prime ribs, most chops, meatloaf, creamed soups and sauces, and salads already coated with dressings.

HOW TO USE *THE DIETER'S COMPLETE GUIDE*

If you are on a restricted diet or if you have decided to limit the amount of calories, carbohydrate, fat, saturated fat, cholesterol, or sodium that you consume, this guide will be invaluable. For each entry you will find the number of calories and quantities of these important substances found in a portion of that food. You can use these values to compare food choices or to moderate your diet.

In comparing food choices, you may find our tables show surprisingly different values for what appear to be similar foods. For example, commercially prepared items often have important nutritional differences from their homemade counterparts. If you take the time to compare foods within a category, you also may identify food substitutes which more nearly satisfy your dietary requirements than do the usual food items. For example, if you are trying to limit cholesterol, you may wish to use an egg substitute in place of whole eggs for your breakfast scrambled eggs. This guide shows that the substitute is lower in cholesterol than the whole eggs. However, if you want to limit your sodium consumption, you may wish to avoid egg substitutes because they are higher in sodium than unsalted whole eggs.

The Dieter's Complete Guide can also help you choose foods to fit the criteria of your particular diet. If you are counting calories or if you have been told by your physician to limit your consumption of a particular substance, such as sodium or cholesterol, to a specific daily amount, the procedure to follow is quite easy. For example, if your physician has prescribed a 1000 milligrams-per-day sodium diet for you, this book will aid you in checking your daily sodium consumption. You can look up the foods you eat and total their sodium contents.

This simple exercise can be very useful in accustoming yourself to a new diet. Use this book to learn to "pace" your consumption to meet your daily goal. And, if you occasionally want to indulge in a food rich in the "forbidden" substance, you can consult the listings to identify other foods low in your restricted constituent and still meet your goal.

The Data. To assemble this book, the Editors of CONSUMER GUIDE® have used the latest government data on food composition and obtained information on brand-name products directly from manufacturers. In preparing the listings, we used the most recent information available. In spite of these efforts and the cooperation of government agencies and numerous food vendors, we were not able to obtain information on all currently sold products or for all constituents of products. The greatest difficulty encountered was in procuring data on cholesterol and saturated fat; in some cases, the sodium values also eluded us. In those instances where data could not be obtained, you will see the abbreviation NA—standing for Not Available. Another abbreviation—Tr.—indicates that only a trace or minute quantity of the substance was detected.

Watch for the alerts. For people whose diet is not medically restricted, there really are no "bad" foods. A nutritionally balanced diet consisting of a variety of foods is healthful. The old rule—Everything in Moderation—still applies. However, for people on restricted diets, there are groups of foods to beware of. For example, persons who must limit salt intake generally should avoid traditionally prepared hams and luncheon meats which are high in sodium. (Nevertheless, not all foods in a particular food group necessarily pose a problem.) In addition, formerly forbidden food groups have been invaded by specially manufactured "dietetic" foods which meet the needs of the growing ranks of people on restricted diets. If you seek variety in your restricted diet, examine the labels of dietetic products to determine whether the particular product is low in the substance you must avoid. We examined many such products, and you will find the results in the listings.

To enable you to make a quick check of the suitability of a particular food to your diet, we have placed in front of certain food items "flag indicators" or "alerts." These alerts—circles for sodium, squares for cholesterol, and stars for sugar—indicate foods whose consumption generally should be limited or avoided by persons who need to restrict their intake of the specific food substance.

By assigning these special indicators, we have developed a system to alert you to foods you will want to limit if you follow a certain dietary restriction. If you are limiting your cholesterol intake, you will want to avoid foods preceded by black squares. If you must limit your sodium intake, beware of foods flagged by a black circle. If you must restrict your sugar intake, take special notice of the foods preceded by black stars.

In general, the foods alerted for cholesterol and sodium are relatively high in the particular constituent, particularly in comparison to (1) other similar foods, (2) comparable serving sizes, or (3) appropriate substitutes. For example, one pat of regular butter does not seem to be particularly high in salt, but it receives a sodium alert because individuals restricting sodium reasonably should use unsalted butter or margarine.

In assigning sugar alerts, a somewhat simpler rationale was used: if any form of "sugar" is an ingredient in the particular food (unless so minimal that its presence is almost negligible), an alert is given to that food.

For certain brand-name foods, we were unable to obtain specific data on sugar, cholesterol, or sodium content (signified by NA), yet we knew you would question whether those foods should be avoided. Hence, when information on a specific brand name item was not available, we checked the ingredients and also sought comparable foods in government data. Based on these two factors, we decided whether or not to assign an alert.

Understanding the Food Descriptions. For every food item, a quantity of food is specified. It may be a weight, volume, serving, or portion. In each case, we have attempted to select the food unit which would be useful in everyday life.

To provide you with information on the widest spectrum of food items available in the American marketplace, we have kept the food descriptions as brief as possible. Thus, in most cases, we have not specified ingredients or recipes. (A few abbreviations are used, the only one of which may be unfamiliar is "w/o" as an abbreviation for "without.") You should be aware that when no specifications are shown, the listing applies to the usual or most common form of the item. Thus, with raw foods, you can assume that no sugar, salt, or other ingredient has been added to the food. With the many "homemade" foods, you can assume that the foods have been prepared according to usual American cooking practices. Unless it is specified, you can assume that a dietetic recipe has not been used. Hence, homemade cakes are flagged with black stars because sugar is a prominent ingredient in the usual recipes, in spite of the fact that there are dietetic cake recipes suitable for individuals who must restrict their sugar intake. Likewise, you should anticipate that the homemade recipes contain the usual salt, fat, and cholesterol.

Information also is given for the many commercial, partially prepared foods which undergo further preparation in the home. Most times, we have given the composition of unprepared foods so that you will see what happens when you omit or substitute certain ingredients. Where useful and appropriate, we show the composition of the prepared food. "Prepared" means that the package directions are followed. For example, if the frozen vegetable package directs you to add butter and salt, a listing designated "prepared" (or boiled, baked, etc.) would include the content of those ingredients.

Beans/Legumes

Food Description	Calories	Carbohydrates (grams)	Fat (grams)	Saturated Fat (grams)	Cholesterol (milligrams)	Sodium (milligrams)
Chickpeas (garbanzos), dry (1 lb.)	1633	276.7	21.8	2.0	0	117
● Garbanzos, *Joan of Arc* (½ cup)	120	19.0	2.0	NA	0	NA
Garbanzos, *Nutradiet* (½ cup)	105	19.0	1.0	Tr.	0	10
Lentils, cooked (1 cup)	212	38.6	0	0	0	26
Lentils, dry (1 cup)	646	114.2	2.1	0	0	57
Peas, dry, split (1 lb.)	1579	284.4	4.5	0	0	181
Peas, dry, split, cooked (1 cup)	230	41.6	0.6	0	0	26
BEANS						
Black/brown/Bayo, raw (1 cup)	678	122.4	3.0	0	0	50
Broad, raw, dry (1 lb.)	1533	264.0	7.7	0	0	36
●★ Butter, *Joan of Arc* (½ cup)	100	17.0	0	0	0	NA
●★ Butter, *Van Camp's* (1 cup)	170	33.0	0	0	0	840
●★ Butter, *Winter Garden* (3.3 oz.)	140	26.0	1.0	Tr.	0	241
● Kidney, dark red, *Van Camp's* (1 cup)	200	39.0	1.0	0	0	790
● Kidney, light red, *Van Camp's* (1 cup)	210	41.0	1.0	0	0	750
Kidney, *Nutradiet* (½ cup)	90	16.0	0	0	0	10
Kidney, red, cooked, no salt (1 cup)	218	39.6	0.9	0	0	6
Kidney, red, raw (1 cup)	635	114.5	2.8	0	0	19
●★■ Lima, baby, butter sauce, frozen, *Green Giant* (1 cup)	200	32.0	4.0	NA	NA	885
● Lima, baby, frozen, *Birds Eye* (3.3 oz.)	120	22.0	1.0	0	0	115
Lima, baby, frozen, *Green Giant* (3½ oz.)	100	19.7	0.5	0	0	49
Lima, mature, cooked, no salt (1 cup)	262	48.6	1.1	0	0	4
Navy, dried (1 cup)	697	125.7	3.3	0	0	39
Navy, dried, cooked, no salt (1 cup)	224	40.3	1.1	0	0	13

Alerts: ● Sodium ★ Sugar ■ Cholesterol

Food Description	Calories	Carbohydrates (grams)	Fat (grams)	Saturated Fat (grams)	Cholesterol (milligrams)	Sodium (milligrams)
Pinto, raw (1 cup)	663	121.0	2.3	0	0	19
Soybean curd (1 lb.)	327	10.9	19.1	2.9	0	32
Soybeans, cooked, no salt (1 cup)	234	19.4	10.3	1.6	0	4
Soybeans, dry (1 cup)	846	70.4	37.2	5.6	0	11
●White, canned (1 cup)	306	58.6	1.3	0	0	862
White, dried (1 lb.)	1542	278.1	7.3	0	0	86
BAKED BEANS						
●★Brown sugar, *Van Camp's* (1 cup)	330	58.0	6.0	NA	NA	800
●★Kidney, red, *B & M* (8 oz.)	330	50.0	7.0	NA	NA	776
●★Kidney, red, New Orleans style, *Van Camp's* (1 cup)	210	39.0	1.0	Tr.	NA	900
●★Molasses brown sugar sauce, old fashioned, *Campbell's* (8 oz.)	290	49.0	5.0	NA	NA	930
●★Vegetarian style, *Van Camp's* (1 cup)	240	49.0	1.0	Tr.	0	1100
●★Vegetarian, tomato sauce, *Libby's* (1 cup)	260	51.0	1.0	Tr.	0	810
●★With pork, *B & M* (8 oz.)	330	49.0	8.0	NA	NA	848
●★With pork, *Campbell's* (8 oz.)	260	43.0	4.0	NA	NA	955
●★With pork, molasses sauce, *Libby's* (1 cup)	280	49.0	4.0	NA	Tr.	515
●★With pork, *Van Camp's* (1 cup)	260	47.0	2.0	NA	NA	1180
●★With pork, tomato sauce, *Libby's* (1 cup)	270	49.0	3.0	NA	Tr.	850

Beverages

ALCOHOLIC BEVERAGES						
Beer						
Augustine (12 oz.)	157	10.6	0	0	0	21
Augustine Light (12 oz.)	96	2.2	0	0	0	14
Beer/4.5% alcohol (12 oz.)	151	13.7	0	0	0	25
Blatz (12 oz.)	150	11.0	0	0	0	22
Budweiser (12 oz.)	150	12.8	0	0	0	14
Busch (12 oz.)	146	12.4	0	0	0	14

Alerts: ● Sodium ★ Sugar ■ Cholesterol

Food Description	Calories	Carbohydrates (grams)	Fat (grams)	Saturated Fat (grams)	Cholesterol (milligrams)	Sodium (milligrams)
Michelob (12 oz.)	163	14.9	0	0	0	14
Michelob Light (12 oz.)	134	12.0	0	0	0	14
Natural Light (12 oz.)	110	5.5	0	0	0	14
Old Milwaukee (12 oz.)	143	13.6	0	0	0	NA
Old Style (12 oz.)	150	11.0	0	0	0	22
Schlitz (12 oz.)	150	13.6	0	0	0	NA
Schlitz Light (12 oz.)	96	5.1	0	0	0	NA
★Cordial, apricot, *Hiram Walker* (1 oz.)	79	8.0	0	0	0	NA
Distilled Spirits						
Bourbon, *Walker's Deluxe, Ten High* (1 jigger)	107	0	0	0	0	Tr.
Brandy, *Walker's* (1 jigger)	99	0	0	0	0	NA
Gin, *London Dry* (1 jigger)	99	0	0	0	0	Tr.
Gin, rum, vodka, whiskey/86-proof (1 jigger)	105	0	0	0	0	Tr.
Gin, rum, vodka, whiskey/90-proof (1 jigger)	110	0	0	0	0	Tr.
Gin, rum, vodka, whiskey/100-proof (1 jigger)	124	0	0	0	0	Tr.
Scotch whiskey, *Thorne* (1 jigger)	107	0	0	0	0	Tr.
Vodka, *Hiram Walker* (1 jigger)	99	0	0	0	0	Tr.
Whiskey, *Canadian Club* (1 jigger)	107	0	0	0	0	Tr.
★Liqueur, amaretto, *Hiram Walker* (1 oz.)	76	8.9	0	0	0	NA
★Liqueur, creme de cacao, white, *Hiram Walker* (1 oz.)	96	13.0	0	0	0	NA
★Liqueur, creme de menthe, *Hiram Walker* (1 oz.)	96	11.8	0	0	0	NA
★Liqueur, triple sec, *Hiram Walker* (1 oz.)	90	10.3	0	0	0	NA
Wine						
Burgundy, hearty, *Gallo* (1 oz.)	23	0.4	0	0	0	Tr.
Burgundy, sparkling, *Paul Masson* (1 oz.)	25	Tr.	0	0	0	Tr.
Champagne, *Paul Masson* (1 oz.)	25	Tr.	0	0	0	Tr.
Cream Sherry, *Livingston* (1 oz.)	40	3.0	0	0	0	Tr.
Dessert/18.8% alcohol (1 oz.)	41	2.3	0	0	0	Tr.
French Colombard, *Gallo* (1 oz.)	21	0.5	0	0	0	Tr.

Alerts: ● Sodium ★ Sugar ■ Cholesterol

Food Description	Calories	Carbohydrates (grams)	Fat (grams)	Saturated Fat (grams)	Cholesterol (milligrams)	Sodium (milligrams)
Port, *Paul Masson* (1 oz.)	47	NA	0	0	0	Tr.
Sauvignon Blanc, *Gallo* (1 oz.)	19	0.2	0	0	0	Tr.
Sherry, *Paul Masson* (1 oz.)	38	NA	0	0	0	Tr.
Table/12.2% alcohol (1 oz.)	25	1.2	0	0	0	Tr.
Vin Rose, *Gallo* (1 oz.)	22	0.6	0	0	0	Tr.
CARBONATED BEVERAGES						
Club soda, *Canada Dry* (8 oz.)	0	0	0	0	0	60
Club soda, *Schweppes* (10 oz.)	0	0	0	0	0	44
Colas						
Canfield's, sugar free (8 oz.)	2	0.2	0	0	0	56
★Coca-Cola (8 oz.)	96	24.0	0	0	0	20
Diet Pepsi-Cola (12 oz.)	1	0	0	0	0	62
Diet-Rite, sugar free (12 oz.)	1	0	0	0	0	37
★Pepsi (8 oz.)	105	26.4	0	0	0	6
Pepsi Light (8 oz.)	1	Tr.	0	0	0	28
RC 100 (12 oz.)	1	0.1	0	0	0	37
★Royal Crown (12 oz.)	156	38.9	0	0	0	1
Tab (8 oz.)	1	0.1	0	0	0	30
★Collins mixer, *Canada Dry* (8 oz.)	80	20.0	0	0	0	17
Diet 7 Up (12 oz.)	4	0	0	0	0	48
★Dr. Pepper (6 oz.)	72	19.0	0	0	0	14
Dr. Pepper, sugar free (6 oz.)	2	0.4	0	0	0	18
Fresca, sugar free (12 oz.)	4	0	0	0	0	61
★Ginger ale, *Canada Dry* (8 oz.)	90	21.0	0	0	0	NA
Ginger ale, *Canada Dry*, sugar free (8 oz.)	2	0	0	0	0	29
★Ginger ale, *Schweppes* (10 oz.)	110	27.1	0	0	0	19
Ginger ale, *Schweppes*, no sugar (6 oz.)	2	0	0	0	0	20
★Grape, *Fanta* (8 oz.)	114	29.0	0	0	0	21
★Grape, *Nehi* (12 oz.)	174	43.6	0	0	0	14
★Orange, *Fanta* (8 oz.)	117	30.0	0	0	0	21
★Orange, *Nehi* (12 oz.)	190	47.5	0	0	0	22
★Quinine water (12 oz.)	113	29.3	0	0	0	NA
Quinine water, sugar free, *Canfield's* (8 oz.)	4	0	0	0	0	32
★Root beer, *A & W* (12 oz.)	170	42.0	0	0	0	61
Root beer, *A & W*, sugar free (12 oz.)	2	Tr.	0	0	0	79
★Root beer, *Barrelhead* (8 oz.)	110	26.0	0	0	0	17

Alerts: ● Sodium ★ Sugar ■ Cholesterol

Food Description	Calories	Carbohydrates (grams)	Fat (grams)	Saturated Fat (grams)	Cholesterol (milligrams)	Sodium (milligrams)
Root beer, *Dad's,* sugar free (12 oz.)	1	0.3	0	0	0	NA
★Root beer, *Fanta* (8 oz.)	103	27.0	0	0	0	23
★*7 Up* (12 oz.)	144	36.0	0	0	0	32
★*Sprite* (8 oz.)	95	24.0	0	0	0	42
Sprite, no sugar (8 oz.)	3	0	0	0	0	42
Strawberry, *Tab* (8 oz.)	2	0	0	0	0	39
★Tonic, *Canada Dry* (8 oz.)	90	22.0	0	0	0	NA
Tonic, *Canada Dry,* low calorie (8 oz.)	4	0	0	0	0	24
★Tonic, *Schweppes* (10 oz.)	110	27.5	0	0	0	7
Tonic, *Schweppes,* no sugar (6 oz.)	1	0	0	0	0	37
COFFEE AND TEA						
Coffee, all grinds, brewed, *Maxwell House* (6 oz.)	2	0	0	0	0	Tr.
Coffee, electric perk, decaffeinated, brewed, *Brim* (6 oz.)	2	0	0	0	0	1
Coffee, freeze dried, prepared, *Tasters Choice* (1 serving)	4	1.0	0	0	0	10
★Coffee, instant, coffee-flavor grain beverage, prepared, *Postum* (6 oz.)	10	2.0	0	0	0	3
●★Coffee, instant drink, *Bavarian Mint* (6 oz.)	10	12.0	1.0	NA	NA	NA
●★Coffee, instant drink, *Cafe Vienna* (6 oz.)	10	11.0	2.0	NA	NA	95
●★Coffee, instant drink, prepared, *Orange Cappuccino* (6 oz.)	60	10.0	2.0	NA	NA	100
●★Coffee, instant drink, prepared, *Toffee Mocha* (6 oz.)	50	13.0	1.0	NA	NA	NA
Coffee, instant, 97% caffeine-free, prepared, *Sanka* (6 oz.)	4	1.0	0	0	0	Tr.
Tea, black rum flavor, brewed, *Lipton* (1 cup)	2	1.0	0	0	0	Tr.
Tea, instant, lemon flavor, prepared, *Lipton* (8 oz.)	4	0	0	0	0	NA
Tea, instant, prepared, *Nestea* (1 serving)	4	1.0	0	0	0	10
★Tea, lemon flavor, canned, *Lemon Tree* (8 oz.)	90	22.0	0	0	0	NA

Alerts: ● Sodium ★ Sugar ■ Cholesterol

Food Description	Calories	Carbohydrates (grams)	Fat (grams)	Saturated Fat (grams)	Cholesterol (milligrams)	Sodium (milligrams)
Tea, lemon flavor, canned, sugar free, *Lemon Tree* (8 oz.)	2	0	0	0	0	NA
Tea mix, lemon flavor, sugar free, *Lemon Tree* (8 oz.)	2	0	0	0	0	NA
★Tea mix, lemon, sweetened, prepared, *Nestea* (1 serving)	70	17.0	0	0	0	10

DIET AND BREAKFAST BEVERAGES

Food Description	Calories	Carbohydrates (grams)	Fat (grams)	Saturated Fat (grams)	Cholesterol (milligrams)	Sodium (milligrams)
●★Diet liquid, butterscotch, *Sego* (10 oz.)	225	34.0	5.0	NA	NA	NA
●★Diet liquid, chocolate, *Slender* (10 oz.)	225	34.0	5.0	NA	NA	515
●★Diet liquid, Dutch chocolate flavor, *Sego* (10 oz.)	225	39.0	3.0	NA	NA	NA
●★Diet liquid, French vanilla, *Sego* (10 oz.)	225	34.0	5.0	NA	NA	NA
●★Diet liquid, strawberry flavor, *Sego* (10 oz.)	225	34.0	5.0	NA	NA	NA
●★Diet liquid, strawberry, *Slender* (10 oz.)	225	34.0	5.0	NA	NA	431
●★Diet liquid, vanilla, *Slender* (10 oz.)	225	34.0	5.0	NA	NA	550
●★Diet mix, chocolate, *Slender* (1 envelope)	113	20.0	1.0	NA	NA	105
●★Diet mix, strawberry flavor, *Sego* (1 oz.)	105	21.0	0	0	NA	NA
●★Diet mix, strawberry, *Slender* (1 envelope)	113	21.0	0	0	NA	104
●★Diet mix, vanilla flavor, *Sego* (1 oz.)	105	21.0	0	0	NA	NA
●★Diet mix, vanilla, *Slender* (1 envelope)	113	21.0	0	0	NA	91
●★Food drink, chocolate, *Nutrament* (12 oz.)	360	52.0	10.0	1.2	6	200
●★Food drink, vanilla, *Nutrament* (12 oz.)	360	52.0	10.0	1.2	6	200

Instant Breakfast Mixes

Food Description	Calories	Carbohydrates (grams)	Fat (grams)	Saturated Fat (grams)	Cholesterol (milligrams)	Sodium (milligrams)
●★Chocolate, *Carnation* (1 envelope)	130	23.0	1.0	NA	NA	136
●★Chocolate malt, *Pillsbury* (1 envelope)	130	26.0	0	0	NA	140
●★Chocolate malt, *Carnation* (1 envelope)	130	22.0	1.0	NA	NA	187

Alerts: ● Sodium ★ Sugar ■ Cholesterol

Food Description	Calories	Carbohydrates (grams)	Fat (grams)	Saturated Fat (grams)	Cholesterol (milligrams)	Sodium (milligrams)
●★Chocolate, *Pillsbury* (1 envelope)	130	26.0	0	0	NA	135
●★Eggnog flavor, *Carnation* (1 envelope)	130	23.0	0	0	NA	196
●★Strawberry, *Carnation* (1 envelope)	130	24.0	0	0	NA	194
●★Strawberry flavor, *Pillsbury* (1 envelope)	130	27.0	0	0	NA	125
●★Vanilla, *Carnation* (1 envelope)	130	24.0	0	0	NA	145
●★Vanilla flavor, *Pillsbury* (1 envelope)	130	27.0	0	0	NA	120
FRUIT AND VEGETABLE DRINKS						
★All flavors, *Hi-C Soft Drinks* (6 oz.)	80	20.0	0	0	0	15
★A.M., *Mott's* (6 oz.)	90	22.0	0	0	0	NA
★Apple-cherry cocktail, *Musselman* (8 oz.)	110	28.0	0	0	0	NA
★Apple-cranberry, *Hi-C* (6 oz.)	90	21.0	Tr.	0	0	Tr.
● Clam and tomato flavor cocktail, *Clamato* (6 oz.)	80	19.0	0	0	0	815
Cranapple, low calorie, *Ocean Spray* (6 oz.)	30	7.0	0	0	0	8
★*Cranapple, Ocean Spray* (6 oz.)	130	32.0	0	0	0	4
★Cranberry juice cocktail, low calorie, *Ocean Spray* (6 oz.)	35	9.0	0	0	0	6
★Cranberry juice cocktail, *Ocean Spray* (6 oz.)	110	26.0	0	0	0	3
★Fruit punch, *Hi-C* (6 oz.)	93	23.0	Tr.	0	0	Tr.
★Fruit punch, low sugar, *Hawaiian Punch* (6 oz.)	30	8.0	0	0	0	NA
●★Fruit punch, red and very berry, *Hawaiian Punch* (6 oz.)	90	22.0	0	0	0	NA
★Grape, *Hi-C* (6 oz.)	89	22.0	Tr.	0	0	Tr.
Grapefruit, low calorie, *Wagner* (6 oz.)	16	4.0	0	0	0	NA
★Grapefruit-orange cocktail, *Musselman* (8 oz.)	90	23.0	0	0	0	NA
★Grapefruit and orange, *Wagner* (6 oz.)	90	21.0	0	0	0	NA
★Lemonade, chilled, *Minute Maid* (6 oz.)	79	18.0	Tr.	0	0	Tr.

Alerts: ● Sodium ★ Sugar ■ Cholesterol

Food Description	Calories	Carbohydrates (grams)	Fat (grams)	Saturated Fat (grams)	Cholesterol (milligrams)	Sodium (milligrams)
★Lemonade, frozen concentrate, prepared, *Minute Maid* (6 oz.)	74	19.6	Tr.	0	0	1
●Lemon-lime and orange, *Gatorade* (8 oz.)	50	14.0	0	0	0	130
★Limeade, frozen concentrate, prepared, *Minute Maid* (6 oz.)	75	20.1	Tr.	0	0	Tr.
★Orange, frozen concentrate, prepared, *Birds Eye Awake* (6 oz.)	80	21.0	0	0	0	10
★Orange, frozen concentrate, prepared, *Birds Eye Orange Plus* (6 oz.)	100	24.0	0	0	0	10
★Orange, *Hi-C* (6 oz.)	92	23.0	Tr.	0	0	58
Orange, low calorie, *Wagner* (6 oz.)	15	3.0	0	0	0	NA
★Orange-pineapple cocktail, *Musselman* (8 oz.)	100	23.0	0	0	0	NA
★Pineapple-grapefruit, *Del Monte* (6 oz.)	90	24.0	0	0	0	45
★Pineapple-orange, *Del Monte* (6 oz.)	90	23.0	0	0	0	10
★Pineapple-pink grapefruit, *Dole* (6 oz.)	101	25.4	0.1	0	0	Tr.
●★Tomato cocktail, *Firehouse Jubilee* (6 oz.)	45	9.0	0	0	0	599
Vegetable juice cocktail, low sodium, *Green Label* (6 oz.)	35	8.0	0	0	0	20
Vegetable juice cocktail, low sodium, *V-8* (6 oz.)	35	8.0	0	0	0	60
●Vegetable juice cocktail, spicy hot, *V-8* (6 oz.)	40	8.0	0	0	0	569
●Vegetable juice cocktail, *V-8* (6 oz.)	35	8.0	0	0	0	555
★Wild berry, *Hi-C* (6 oz.)	88	22.0	Tr.	0	0	5

FRUIT AND VEGETABLE JUICES

Food Description	Calories	Carbohydrates (grams)	Fat (grams)	Saturated Fat (grams)	Cholesterol (milligrams)	Sodium (milligrams)
Apple, *Minute Maid* (6 oz.)	100	24.0	Tr.	0	0	2
Apple, *Mott's* (6 oz.)	80	19.0	0	0	0	10
Apple, *Musselman* (6 oz.)	80	21.0	0	0	0	NA
Apricot nectar, *Del Monte* (6 oz.)	100	26.0	0	0	0	10
Apricot-pineapple nectar, *Blue Label* (6 oz.)	35	12.0	0	0	0	NA

Alerts: ● Sodium ★ Sugar ■ Cholesterol

Food Description	Calories	Carbohydrates (grams)	Fat (grams)	Saturated Fat (grams)	Cholesterol (milligrams)	Sodium (milligrams)
Blackberry, canned (1 cup)	91	19.1	1.5	0	0	2
● Carrot, *Eveready* (6 oz.)	70	16.0	0	0	0	200
Grape, *Welch's* (6 oz.)	120	30.0	0	0	0	NA
Grape, canned (1 cup)	167	42.0	0	0	0	5
★ Grape, frozen concentrate, sweetened, prepared, *Minute Maid* (6 oz.)	99	25.0	Tr.	0	0	2
Grapefruit, *Minute Maid* (6 oz.)	75	17.0	0.1	0	0	2
★ Grapefruit, canned sweetened (1 cup)	133	32.0	0.3	0	0	3
Grapefruit, chilled, *Minute Maid* (6 oz.)	75	18.1	Tr.	0	0	2
Grapefruit, dehydrated (1 oz.)	107	25.6	0.3	0	0	2
Grapefruit, Florida (1 cup)	91	21.6	0.2	0	0	3
Grapefruit, frozen concentrate, prepared, *Minute Maid* (6 oz.)	75	18.3	Tr.	0	0	Tr.
★ Grapefruit, frozen concentrate, sweetened, prepared (1 cup)	117	28.3	0.2	0	0	3
Grapefruit, *Ocean Spray* (6 oz.)	60	15.0	0	0	0	7
Grapefruit/orange, frozen concentrate, prepared (1 cup)	109	26.0	0.2	0	0	0
Lemon, bottled, reconstituted, natural strength, *Realemon* (2 Tbsp.)	6	2.0	0	0	0	10
Lemon, frozen concentrate, prepared, *Minute Maid* (6 oz.)	40	13.2	Tr.	0	0	2
Lime, fresh or canned (1 Tbsp.)	4	1.4	0	0	0	Tr.
Orange (1 cup)	112	25.8	0.5	0	0	3
★ Orange, canned, sweetened (6 oz.)	97	22.8	0.4	0	0	2
Orange, chilled, *Minute Maid* (6 oz.)	83	19.7	0.1	0	0	1
Orange, dehydrated (1 oz.)	108	25.2	0.5	0	0	2
Orange, *Del Monte* (6 oz.)	70	18.0	0	0	0	10
Orange, frozen concentrate, prepared, *Minute Maid* (6 oz.)	86	20.5	Tr.	0	0	1
Orange, frozen concentrate, prepared, *Snow Crop* (6 oz.)	86	20.5	Tr.	0	0	2

Alerts: ● Sodium ★ Sugar ■ Cholesterol

Food Description	Calories	Carbohydrates (grams)	Fat (grams)	Saturated Fat (grams)	Cholesterol (milligrams)	Sodium (milligrams)
Orange-grapefruit, *Del Monte* (6 oz.)	80	19.0	0	0	0	10
Peach nectar, *Del Monte* (6 oz.)	100	27.0	0	0	0	10
Pear nectar, *Del Monte* (6 oz.)	110	30.0	0	0	0	10
Pineapple, *Dole* (6 oz. can)	103	25.4	0.2	0	0	2
Pineapple, frozen concentrate, prepared (1 cup)	130	32.0	0	0	0	3
Pineapple, *S & W* (6 oz.)	100	25.0	0	0	0	Tr.
Prune, *Sunsweet* (6 oz.)	140	33.0	0	0	0	14
Prune, *Super Mott's* (6 oz.)	140	34.0	0	0	0	NA
Prune, with pulp, *Mott's* (6 oz.)	120	30.0	0	0	0	NA
• Sauerkraut, canned (1 cup)	24	5.6	0	0	0	1904
Tangelo (1 cup)	101	24.0	0.2	0	0	3
Tangerine, canned (6 oz.)	80	18.9	0.4	0	0	2
Tangerine, frozen concentrate, prepared (1 cup)	114	26.8	0.5	0	0	2
• Tomato, *Libby* (6 oz.)	35	8.0	0	0	0	455
• Tomato, *Del Monte* (6 oz.)	35	8.0	0	0	0	480
Tomato, low sodium, *Featherweight* (6 oz.)	35	8.0	0	0	0	20
Tomato, low sodium, *Green Label* (6 oz.)	35	8.0	0	0	0	20
• Tomato, *Stokely* (8 oz.)	40	9.0	0	0	0	660

FRUIT DRINK MIXES

Food Description	Calories	Carbohydrates (grams)	Fat (grams)	Saturated Fat (grams)	Cholesterol (milligrams)	Sodium (milligrams)
All flavors, unsweetened, prepared, *Kool-Aid* (8 oz.)	2	Tr.	0	0	0	0
★ Cherry flavor, prepared, *Kool-Aid* (8 oz.)	100	25.0	0	0	0	Tr.
Cherry flavor, unsweetened, prepared, *Wyler's* (8 oz.)	2	1.0	0	0	0	NA
Cherry, fruit punch, grape and lemonade flavor, low calorie, prepared, *Sweet 'N Low* (1 cup)	40	9.0	0	0	0	25
★ Cherry, grape, lemonade punch, orange, red punch and strawberry flavor, prepared, *Hawaiian Punch* (8 oz.)	100	25.0	0	0	0	NA
★ Cranberry-apple and orange flavor, prepared, *Sweet 'N Low* (½ cup)	40	9.0	1.0	0	0	36
★ Grape flavor, prepared, *Hi-C* (6 oz.)	68	17.0	0	0	0	42

Alerts: • Sodium ★ Sugar ■ Cholesterol

Food Description	Calories	Carbohydrates (grams)	Fat (grams)	Saturated Fat (grams)	Cholesterol (milligrams)	Sodium (milligrams)
★Grape flavor, prepared, *Tang* (4 oz.)	60	15.0	0	0	0	0
★Grapefruit flavor, prepared, *Tang* (4 oz.)	50	13.0	0	0	0	7
★Grape, raspberry and strawberry, sweetened, prepared, *Kool-Aid* (8 oz.)	90	23.0	0	0	0	Tr.
★Lemonade and pink lemonade, sweetened, *Kool-Aid* (8 oz.)	90	22.0	0	0	0	Tr.
Lemonade flavor, low calorie, prepared, *Lemon Tree* (8 oz.)	8	2.0	0	0	0	NA
★Lemonade flavor, prepared, *Country Time* (8 oz.)	90	22.0	0	0	0	60
★Lemonade flavor, prepared, *Wyler's* (8 oz.)	90	22.0	0	0	0	NA
Lemonade flavor, unsweetened, prepared, *Wyler's* (8 oz.)	4	1.0	0	0	0	NA
★Lemonade, prepared, *Lemon Tree* (8 oz.)	90	23.0	0	0	0	NA
●★Lemon-lime and orange flavor, prepared, *Gatorade* (8 oz.)	60	15.0	0	0	0	130
★Lime flavor, prepared, *Country Time* (8 oz.)	90	22.0	0	0	0	50
★Orange flavor, prepared, *Hi-C* (6 oz.)	68	17.0	0	0	0	1
★Orange flavor, prepared, *Tang* (4 oz.)	60	15.0	0	0	0	7
★Orange, sweetened, prepared, *Kool-Aid* (8 oz.)	90	23.0	0	0	0	35
★Punch, prepared, *Hi-C* (6 oz.)	72	18.0	Tr.	0	0	1
★Strawberry, prepared, *Hi-C* (6 oz.)	68	17.0	Tr.	0	0	43
MILK AND MILK BEVERAGES						
★Chocolate flavor, *Nestle Quik* (2 Tbsp.)	90	19.0	1.0	Tr.	0	35
●★Chocolate flavor, *PDQ* (3-4 tsp)	65	14.0	1.0	Tr.	0	NA
●★Cocoa mix (4 heaping tsp.)	102	20.1	0.8	0.5	2	149
●★Cocoa mix, hot, *Lite, Swiss Miss* (¾ oz.)	70	17.0	0	0	0	109
●Cocoa mix, hot, reduced calorie, *Alba '66* (1 envelope)	60	11.0	1.0	NA	0	85

Alerts: ● Sodium ★ Sugar ■ Cholesterol

Food Description	Calories	Carbohydrates (grams)	Fat (grams)	Saturated Fat (grams)	Cholesterol (milligrams)	Sodium (milligrams)
●★Cocoa mix, instant, milk chocolate, *Carnation* (1 oz.)	112	22.0	1.2	NA	NA	111
●★Cocoa mix, low calorie, rich chocolate, *Carnation* (1 envelope)	70	15.0	0	0	NA	102
●★Cocoa mix, low calorie, with marshmallows, *Carnation* (1 envelope)	70	15.0	0	0	NA	123
●★Cocoa mix, *Ovaltine* (1 oz.)	120	22.0	3.0	NA	NA	183
●★Cocoa mix, *Nestle* (1 oz.)	110	22.0	1.0	Tr.	Tr.	145
●★Cocoa mix, reduced calorie, *Ovaltine* (0.7 oz.)	80	15.0	2.0	NA	NA	135
●★Cocoa mix, with marshmallows, *Carnation* (1 oz.)	109	22.0	1.2	Tr.	Tr.	114
Cocoa powder, *Hershey* (⅓ cup)	120	13.0	4.0	NA	0	5
●★Eggnog flavor, *PDQ* (2 heaping Tbsp.)	113	27.5	0.4	Tr.	Tr.	NA
★Flavoring syrup, chocolate, *Bosco* (1 Tbsp.)	50	13.0	0	0	NA	25
●★Flavoring powder, chocolate, *Ovaltine* (¾ oz.)	80	16.0	1.0	Tr.	0	146
Milk						
● Buttermilk, from skim milk (1 cup)	88	12.5	0.2	0	5	319
●★■Chocolate, commercial (1 cup)	213	27.5	8.5	4.7	32	118
●★Chocolate, commercial, skim, 2% fat added (1 cup)	190	27.2	5.8	3.2	20	115
●★■Cocoa, homemade, hot (1 cup)	243	27.2	11.5	6.3	35	128
● Dry, nonfat, instant, chocolate, reconstituted, *Alba* (1 cup)	80	13.0	1.0	Tr.	5	116
●★■Condensed, sweetened (1 cup)	982	166.2	26.6	14.7	104	343
●★■Condensed, sweetened, *Borden's Eagle* (⅓ cup)	320	52.0	9.0	NA	NA	NA
● Dry, nonfat, instant, *Pet* (5 tsp.)	80	12.0	1.0	Tr.	NA	NA
● Dry, nonfat, instant, reconstituted, *Alba* (1 cup)	80	12.0	0	Tr.	5	130
● Dry, nonfat, instant, reconstituted, *Carnation* (1 cup)	80	12.0	0.2	Tr.	NA	124
●★■Eggnog (1 cup)	342	34.4	19.0	11.3	149	138

Alerts: ● Sodium ★ Sugar ■ Cholesterol

Food Description	Calories	Carbohydrates (grams)	Fat (grams)	Saturated Fat (grams)	Cholesterol (milligrams)	Sodium (milligrams)
●■ Eggnog, canned, *Borden* (4 oz.)	160	16.0	9.0	NA	NA	NA
●■ Evaporated (1 cup)	345	24.4	19.9	10.9	78	297
●■ Evaporated, *Carnation* (½ cup)	172	12.4	9.5	NA	NA	129
● Evaporated, filled, *Dairymate* (½ cup)	150	12.0	8.0	1.0	5	NA
● Evaporated, low fat, *Carnation* (4 oz.)	110	12.0	3.0	NA	NA	138
● Evaporated, skim, canned (½ cup)	99	14.5	0.3	0.2	5	147
● Evaporated, skim, *Pet 99* (½ cup)	100	14.0	0	0	NA	NA
● Low fat, 1% fat (1 cup)	119	13.6	2.9	1.8	10	143
● Low fat, 2% nonfat milk solids added (1 cup)	121	11.7	4.7	2.9	18	122
●★■ Malted, dry (3 round tsp.)	116	20.1	2.4	1.4	31	125
★■ Malted, instant, chocolate, *Carnation* (3 heaping tsp.)	85	18.0	1.0	NA	NA	47
●★■ Malted, instant, *Carnation* (3 heaping tsp.)	90	15.6	1.7	NA	NA	98
●★■ Milkshake, thick, chocolate (10.6 oz. container)	356	63.5	8.1	5.0	32	333
●★■ Milkshake, thick, vanilla (11 oz. container)	350	55.6	9.5	5.9	37	299
● Skim (1 cup)	88	12.5	0.2	0	5	127
●■ Whole, 3.7% fat (1 cup)	157	11.4	8.9	5.6	35	119
● Shake mix, chocolate, reduced calorie, *Alba '77 Fit 'N Frosty* (1 envelope)	70	11.0	1.0	Tr.	5	160
● Shake mix, strawberry, reduced calorie, *Alba '77 Fit 'N Frosty* (1 envelope)	70	11.0	0	0	5	180
● Shake mix, vanilla, reduced calorie, *Alba '77 Fit 'N Frosty* (1 envelope)	70	12.0	0	0	5	195

Alerts: ● Sodium ★ Sugar ■ Cholesterol

Biscuits, Rolls, and Muffins

Food Description	Calories	Carbohydrates (grams)	Fat (grams)	Saturated Fat (grams)	Cholesterol (milligrams)	Sodium (milligrams)
BISCUITS						
• Baking powder, dinner, *Tenderflake* (2 biscuits)	110	15.0	4.0	NA	NA	350
• Baking powder, homemade, with self-rising flour (1 oz. biscuit)	105	13.0	4.9	1.2	0	187
• Baking powder, prebaked, *1869 Brand* (2 biscuits)	200	23.0	10.0	NA	NA	555
• Buttermilk, *Big Country*, Pillsbury (2 biscuits)	180	30.0	5.0	NA	NA	720
• Buttermilk, dinner, *Tenderflake* (2 biscuits)	110	15.0	4.0	NA	NA	350
• Buttermilk, *1869 Brand* (2 biscuits)	200	27.0	9.0	NA	NA	590
• Buttermilk, extra rich, *Hungry Jack* (2 biscuits)	130	18.0	6.0	NA	NA	410
• Buttermilk, *Fluffy, Hungry Jack* (2 biscuits)	200	24.0	10.0	NA	NA	605
• Buttermilk, mix, *Bisquick* (½ cup)	240	38.0	8.0	NA	NA	700
• Buttermilk, mix, *Jiffy* (1 oz.)	115	18.7	3.3	NA	NA	NA
• Buttermilk, *Oven Ready*, Ballard (2 biscuits)	100	20.0	1.0	Tr.	NA	600
• Buttermilk, *Pillsbury* (2 biscuits)	100	20.0	1.0	Tr.	NA	430
• Buttermilk, prebaked, *1869 Brand* (2 biscuits)	200	23.0	11.0	NA	NA	565
• *Butter Tastin, 1869 Brand* (2 biscuits)	200	27.0	9.0	NA	NA	590
• *Country Style, Pillsbury* (2 biscuits)	100	20.0	1.0	Tr.	NA	430
• *Flaky, Hungry Jack* (2 biscuits)	180	23.0	9.0	NA	NA	580
• Mix, dry (1 cup)	543	87.9	16.1	3.9	0	1664
• *Oven Ready, Ballard* (2 biscuits)	100	20.0	1.0	Tr.	NA	600
• *Pillsbury Prize* (2 biscuits)	130	19.0	5.0	NA	NA	465
• *Wonder* (2 biscuits)	210	34.0	6.0	NA	5	375

Alerts: • Sodium ★ Sugar ■ Cholesterol

Food Description	Calories	Carbohydrates (grams)	Fat (grams)	Saturated Fat (grams)	Cholesterol (milligrams)	Sodium (milligrams)
CORNBREAD						
●★■ Mix, *Aunt Jemima* (⅙ package)	200	33.0	6.0	NA	NA	NA
●★■ Mix, *Ballard* (⅛ package)	120	24.0	2.0	NA	NA	695
●★■ Mix, dry, *Dromedary* (3 Tbsp.)	110	18.0	4.0	NA	NA	NA
●★■ Muffin, mix, dry, *Betty Crocker* (1/12 package)	140	24.0	4.0	NA	NA	300
●★■ Muffin, mix, dry, *Dromedary* (3½ Tbsp.)	120	20.0	4.0	NA	NA	NA
●★■ Muffin, mix, dry, *Jiffy* (⅛ package)	127	21.7	3.6	NA	NA	NA
●★■ Muffin, mix, prepared (1 muffin)	130	20.0	4.2	1.2	23	192
●★■ Muffin, *Morton Doughnut Shop* (1.7 oz. muffin)	130	20.0	4.0	NA	14	280
●★■ Muffin, *Pepperidge Farm* (1 muffin)	140	21.0	5.0	NA	NA	345
●★■ Muffin, whole ground, homemade (1 muffin)	115	17.0	4.1	1.2	22	198
●★■ *Pepperidge Farm* (1 oz. piece)	110	21.0	1.0	Tr.	NA	518
●★ Pone, homemade (2.1 oz. piece)	122	21.7	2.7	0.9	2	238
●★■ Southern style, homemade with degermed meal (2.9 oz. piece)	186	28.8	5.0	1.3	58	490
●★■ Southern style, homemade with whole-ground meal (2.75 oz. piece)	161	22.7	5.6	1.4	60	490
●★■ Spoonbread, homemade (1 cup)	468	40.6	27.4	8.7	293	1156
MUFFINS						
●★■ Blueberry, homemade (1 muffin)	112	16.8	3.7	1.1	33	253
●★ Blueberry, mix, *Betty Crocker* (1/12 package)	100	18.0	3.0	Tr.	NA	145
●★ Blueberry, mix, *Duncan Hines* (1/12 package)	100	17.0	3.0	0.7	0	180
●★■ Blueberry, *Morton Doughnut Shop* (1 muffin)	120	23.0	3.0	NA	9	130
●★■ Blueberry, *Pepperidge Farm* (1 muffin)	130	22.0	4.0	NA	NA	389
●★ Blueberry round, *Morton Doughnut Shop* (1 round)	110	21.0	3.0	NA	14	180
●★ Bran date, mix, *Jiffy* (⅛ package)	104	17.4	3.1	NA	NA	NA
●★■ Bran, homemade (1 muffin)	104	17.2	3.9	1.2	41	179

Alerts: ● Sodium ★ Sugar ■ Cholesterol

Food Description	Calories	Carbohydrates (grams)	Fat (grams)	Saturated Fat (grams)	Cholesterol (milligrams)	Sodium (milligrams)
●★■ Cinnamon-apple, *Pepperidge Farm* (1 muffin)	140	27.0	2.0	NA	NA	NA
●★ English, *Bays* (2 oz. muffin)	144	24.0	2.0	NA	NA	NA
●★ English, cinnamon/raisin, *Pepperidge Farm* (1 muffin)	150	28.0	2.0	NA	NA	627
●★ English, natural grain, *Newly Weds* (2.5 oz. muffin)	170	33.0	1.0	Tr.	0	NA
●★ English, *Newly Weds* (2½ oz. muffin)	160	29.0	1.0	Tr.	0	NA
●★ English, *Pepperidge Farm* (1 muffin)	140	27.0	1.0	Tr.	NA	633
●★ English, raisin cinnamon, *Newly Weds* (2½ oz. muffin)	171	35.0	2.0	NA	NA	NA
●★ English, sour dough, *Newly Weds* (2.5 oz. muffin)	160	33.0	1.0	Tr.	0	NA
●★ English, *Thomas* (1 muffin)	130	27.0	1.0	Tr.	NA	215
●★ English, *Wonder* (2 oz. muffin)	130	26.0	1.0	Tr.	0	290
●★■ Homemade (1 muffin)	118	16.9	4.0	1.0	21	176
●★■ Plain, *Pepperidge Farm* (1 muffin)	140	27.0	2.0	NA	NA	NA
●★■ Raisin bran, *Pepperidge Farm* (1 muffin)	130	21.0	5.0	NA	NA	180
●★■ Raisin round, *Wonder* (1 round)	150	28.0	3.0	NA	NA	230
●★ Sour dough, *Wonder* (1 muffin)	130	27.0	1.0	Tr.	0	290
ROLLS						
● Cloverleaf (1 oz. roll)	84	15.0	1.6	0.4	2	143
● Crescent, *Ballard* (2 rolls)	190	26.0	8.0	NA	NA	560
● Crescent, *Pillsbury* (2 rolls)	190	25.0	10.0	NA	NA	760
● Dinner, bakery style, frozen, *Pillsbury* (1 roll)	90	18.0	1.0	Tr.	NA	295
● Dinner, *Butterflake, Pillsbury* (1 roll)	110	17.0	3.0	NA	NA	445
● Dinner, *Home Pride* (2 rolls)	180	27.0	6.0	NA	5	265
● Dinner, *Pepperidge Farm* (2 rolls)	120	20.0	4.0	NA	NA	180
● Dough, frozen (1 oz. roll)	76	13.4	1.4	0.3	1	137
● Finger, *Pepperidge Farm* (3 rolls)	180	27.0	5.0	NA	NA	252
● Frankfurter, *Pepperidge Farm* (1 roll)	120	20.0	2.0	NA	NA	205
● French, *Wonder* (2 rolls)	170	27.0	5.0	NA	5	300
● *Half and Half, Wonder* (2 rolls)	170	26.0	5.0	NA	5	145
● Hamburger (1.4 oz. roll)	119	21.2	2.2	0.5	2	202

Alerts: ● Sodium ★ Sugar ■ Cholesterol

Food Description	Calories	Carbohydrates (grams)	Fat (grams)	Saturated Fat (grams)	Cholesterol (milligrams)	Sodium (milligrams)
• Hamburger, *Pepperidge Farm* (1 roll)	120	19.0	3.0	NA	NA	201
• Hard (0.9 oz. roll)	78	14.9	0.8	0.2	1	156
• Hard, Kaiser (1.8 oz. roll)	156	29.8	1.6	0.4	2	312
• *Hearth, Pepperidge Farm* (2 rolls)	110	20.0	2.0	NA	NA	118
• Hoagie or submarine (5 oz. roll)	391	74.8	4.1	0.9	4	783
• Hoagie, *Wonder* (1 roll)	460	82.0	8.0	NA	5	870
• *Home Baked, Wonder* (2 rolls)	170	26.0	5.0	NA	5	230
• Hot dog (2 rolls)	242	43.0	4.5	1.1	5	411
• Parker house, *Pepperidge Farm* (3 rolls)	170	27.0	5.0	NA	NA	273
• Wheat, bakery style, *Pillsbury* (1 roll)	90	16.0	1.0	Tr.	NA	295

Breads

Food Description	Calories	Carbohydrates (grams)	Fat (grams)	Saturated Fat (grams)	Cholesterol (milligrams)	Sodium (milligrams)
• Crumbs, dry, grated (1 cup)	392	73.4	4.6	1.1	5	736
• Crumbs, seasoned, *Contadina* (1 Tbsp.)	50	10.0	0	0	NA	397
• Crumbs, soft (1 cup)	121	22.7	1.4	0.3	1	228
• Cubes, white, soft (1 cup)	81	15.2	1.0	0.2	1	152
• French (1 thick slice)	101	19.4	1.0	0.2	1	203
• French, brown/serve, *Pepperidge Farm* (2 oz.)	150	27.0	3.0	NA	NA	415
• French, *Wonder* (2 slices)	150	27.0	2.0	NA	0	300
• Health nut, *Brownberry* (2 slices)	170	30.0	3.0	NA	NA	405
• Italian (1 thick slice)	83	16.9	0.2	0	0	176
• Italian, brown/serve, *Pepperidge Farm* (2 oz.)	150	28.0	3.0	NA	NA	405
• ★ Raisin (1 slice)	65	13.4	0.7	0.2	1	91
• ★ Raisin cinnamon, *Brownberry* (2 slices)	170	33.0	2.0	NA	0	320
• ★ Raisin nut, *Brownberry* (2 slices)	190	29.0	6.0	NA	0	235

Alerts: • Sodium ★ Sugar ■ Cholesterol

Food Description	Calories	Carbohydrates (grams)	Fat (grams)	Saturated Fat (grams)	Cholesterol (milligrams)	Sodium (milligrams)
★Raisin, *Pepperidge Farm* (2 slices)	150	26.0	3.0	NA	NA	149
•*Roman Meal* (2 slices)	140	27.0	2.0	NA	5	320
• Rye, American (1 slice)	61	13.0	0.3	0.3	0	139
• Rye, *Beefsteak* (2 slices)	150	27.0	2.0	NA	5	330
• Rye, extra thin sliced, *Brownberry* (2 slices)	130	24.0	1.0	Tr.	0	260
• Rye, pumpernickel (1 slice)	79	17.0	0.4	0.3	0	182
• Rye, seedless, *Pepperidge Farm* (2 slices)	160	29.0	2.0	NA	NA	300
• Sour dough, *DiCarlo* (2 slices)	140	27.0	1.0	Tr.	0	290
Taco shell, *Azteca* (0.4 oz.)	51	7.7	1.8	0	0	NA
Taco shell, *Ortega* (1 shell)	50	8.0	2.0	0	0	0
• Vienna (1 slice)	72	13.9	0.8	0.2	1	145
• Wheatberry, *Home Pride* (2 slices)	140	25.0	2.0	NA	0	280
• Wheat, cracked (1 slice)	66	13.0	0.5	0.1	1	132
• Wheat, cracked, *Pepperidge Farm* (2 slices)	140	26.0	2.0	NA	NA	314
• Wheat, cracked, *Wonder* (2 slices)	150	27.0	2.0	NA	5	300
• Wheat, *Fresh Horizons* (2 slices)	100	19.0	1.0	Tr.	0	305
• Wheat, *Hollywood Dark* (2 slices)	140	25.0	2.0	NA	5	375
• Wheat, *Fresh/Natural* (2 slices)	140	27.0	2.0	NA	0	275
• Wheat, *Hollywood Light* (2 slices)	140	26.0	2.0	NA	5	335
• Wheat, *Pepperidge Farm* (2 slices)	190	35.0	3.0	NA	NA	405
• Wheat, whole (1 slice)	61	11.9	0.8	0.2	1	132
•★Wheat, whole, honey prune, *Brownberry* (2 slices)	150	31.0	1.0	Tr.	0	350
• Wheat, whole, *Pepperidge Farm* (2 slices)	140	24.0	3.0	NA	NA	214
• Wheat, whole, *Wonder* (2 slices)	140	24.0	2.0	NA	5	375
• Wheat, *Wonder* (2 slices)	150	27.0	2.0	NA	5	310
• White (1 slice)	77	14.3	0.9	0.2	1	144
• White, *Brownberry* (2 slices)	150	31.0	1.0	Tr.	NA	355
• White, buttertop, *Home Pride* (2 slices)	150	26.0	3.0	NA	5	305
• White, light, *Butternut* (1 slice)	55	11.0	0.5	Tr.	5	NA
White, low-sodium, *Wonder* (2 slices)	140	27.0	2.0	NA	5	6

Alerts: • Sodium ★ Sugar ■ Cholesterol

Food Description	Calories	Carbohydrates (grams)	Fat (grams)	Saturated Fat (grams)	Cholesterol (milligrams)	Sodium (milligrams)
• White, reduced calorie, *Fresh Horizons* (2 slices)	100	19.0	1.0	Tr.	0	NA
• White, sandwich, *Pepperidge Farm* (2 slices)	130	23.0	3.0	NA	NA	260
• White with buttermilk, *Wonder* (2 slices)	150	27.0	2.0	NA	5	345
• Whole bran, *Brownberry* (2 slices)	150	30.0	1.0	Tr.	0	395

CROUTONS AND STUFFINGS

Food Description	Calories	Carbohydrates (grams)	Fat (grams)	Saturated Fat (grams)	Cholesterol (milligrams)	Sodium (milligrams)
• Croutons, cheese garlic, *Pepperidge Farm* (1 oz.)	140	13.0	9.0	NA	NA	276
• Croutons, onion garlic, *Pepperidge Farm* (1 oz.)	130	16.0	6.0	NA	NA	272
• Croutons, plain, *Pepperidge Farm* (1 oz.)	140	20.0	5.0	NA	NA	295
• Croutons, seasoned, *Pepperidge Farm* (1 oz.)	140	19.0	5.0	NA	NA	519
•★ Stuffing, bread, dry (8 oz. package)	842	164.3	8.6	2.0	9	3021
•★■ Stuffing, bread, prepared, moist (1 cup)	416	39.4	25.6	13.1	132	1008
•★ Stuffing, chicken, *Stove Top* (⅙ package)	110	21.0	1.0	Tr.	NA	550
•★ Stuffing, herb, *Kellogg Croutettes* ⁷⁄₁₀ oz.)	70	14.0	0	0	NA	260
•★ Stuffing, herb, *Pepperidge Farm* (1 oz.)	110	23.0	1.0	Tr.	NA	491
•★ Stuffing, pork, *Stove Top* (⅙ package)	110	20.0	1.0	Tr.	NA	570
•★ Stuffing, seasoned, *Pepperidge Farm* (1 oz.)	100	20.0	1.0	Tr.	NA	414
•★ Stuffing, with rice, dry, *Stove Top* (1 serving)	110	23.0	1.0	Tr.	NA	495

Alerts: • Sodium ★ Sugar ■ Cholesterol

Cakes and Icings

Food Description	Calories	Carbohydrates (grams)	Fat (grams)	Saturated Fat (grams)	Cholesterol (milligrams)	Sodium (milligrams)
CAKES						
●★Angelfood, homemade (1/12 cake)	161	36.1	0.1	0	0	169
●★■ Apple 'n cream torte, frozen, *Sara Lee* (1/8 cake)	203	26.2	10.2	NA	NA	146
●★■ Banana, frozen, *Sara Lee* (1/8 cake)	175	26.8	6.9	NA	NA	154
●★■ Banana supreme, frozen, *Pepperidge Farm* (2.9 oz. piece)	280	40.0	12.0	NA	NA	147
●★■ Boston creme supreme, frozen, *Pepperidge Farm* (2.9 oz. piece)	270	43.0	10.0	NA	NA	165
●★■ Carrot, frozen, *Sara Lee* (1/8 cake)	153	18.9	7.8	NA	NA	125
●★■ Cheesecake, cherry, frozen, *Morton's Great Little Dessert* (6 oz. piece)	460	47.0	27.0	NA	106	350
●★■ Cheesecake, cream, frozen, *Morton's Great Little Dessert* (6 oz. piece)	480	42.0	32.0	NA	116	350
●★■ Cheesecake, pineapple, frozen, *Morton's Great Little Dessert* (6 oz. piece)	460	48.0	27.0	NA	106	355
●★■ Cheesecake, strawberry, frozen, *Morton's Great Little Dessert* (6 oz. piece)	470	50.0	27.0	NA	106	350
●★■ Chocolate Bavarian, frozen, *Sara Lee* (1/8 cake)	285	20.2	22.6	NA	NA	78
●★■ Chocolate/chocolate icing, homemade (1/12 layer cake)	365	55.2	16.2	6.4	48	233
●★■ Chocolate, frozen, *Sara Lee* (1/8 cake)	185	28.1	8.9	NA	NA	168
●★■ Chocolate fudge, frozen, *Pepperidge Farm* (1.7 oz. piece)	180	25.0	9.0	NA	NA	166

Alerts: ● Sodium ★ Sugar ■ Cholesterol

Food Description	Calories	Carbohydrates (grams)	Fat (grams)	Saturated Fat (grams)	Cholesterol (milligrams)	Sodium (milligrams)
●★■ Chocolate pound, frozen, *Sara Lee* (¹/₁₀ cake)	122	14.5	6.4	NA	NA	134
●★■ Chocolate/white icing, homemade (¹/₁₂ layer cake)	362	58.0	14.3	5.4	47	229
●★■ Coconut, frozen, *Pepperidge Farm* (1.7 oz. piece)	180	26.0	9.0	NA	NA	140
●★■ Cream cheese, blueberry, frozen, *Sara Lee* (¹/₆ cake)	233	35.3	8.5	NA	NA	175
●★■ Cream cheese, frozen, *Sara Lee* (¹/₆ cake)	231	25.9	11.9	NA	NA	161
●★■ Devil's food, frozen, *Pepperidge Farm* (1.7 oz. piece)	180	26.0	8.0	NA	NA	166
★ Fruitcake, dark, homemade (1 slice)	57	9.0	2.3	0.5	7	23
●★■ German chocolate, frozen, *Pepperidge Farm* (1.7 oz. piece)	160	24.0	6.0	NA	NA	105
●★■ German chocolate, frozen, *Sara Lee* (¹/₈ cake)	172	19.3	9.6	NA	NA	133
●★■ Golden layer, frozen, *Pepperidge Farm* (1.7 oz. piece)	180	25.0	9.0	NA	NA	142
●★■ Lemon coconut supreme, frozen, *Pepperidge Farm* (3 oz. piece)	280	42.0	11.0	NA	NA	186
●★■ Pound, chocolate swirl, frozen, *Sara Lee* (¹/₁₀ cake)	130	17.9	5.7	NA	NA	116
●★■ Pound, frozen, *Sara Lee* (¹/₁₀ cake)	125	14.2	6.9	NA	NA	104
●★■ Pound, homemade (½″ slice)	119	15.9	5.4	1.4	44	51
●★■ Sponge, homemade (¹/₁₂ cake)	196	35.7	3.8	1.9	162	110
●★■ Strawberry cream supreme, frozen, *Pepperidge Farm* (2 oz. piece)	180	28.0	7.0	NA	NA	78
●★■ Vanilla, frozen, *Pepperidge Farm* (1.7 oz. piece)	190	27.0	8.0	NA	NA	143
●★■ Walnut supreme, frozen, *Pepperidge Farm* (2 oz. piece)	240	26.0	14.0	NA	NA	141
●★ White/white icing, homemade, (¹/₁₂ layer cake)	390	65.4	13.4	4.2	8	243
●★■ Yellow/chocolate icing, homemade (¹/₁₂ layer cake)	365	60.4	13.0	4.6	44	208

Alerts: ● Sodium ★ Sugar ■ Cholesterol

Food Description	Calories	Carbohydrates (grams)	Fat (grams)	Saturated Fat (grams)	Cholesterol (milligrams)	Sodium (milligrams)
CAKE MIXES						
●★ Angel food, chocolate, *Betty Crocker* (¹/₁₂ package)	140	32.0	0	0	0	275
●★ Angel food, *Duncan Hines Deluxe II* (¹/₁₂ package)	140	30.0	0	0	0	130
●★ Banana flavor, *Duncan Hines Deluxe II* (¹/₁₂ package)	190	34.0	5.0	NA	NA	240
●★ Banana flavor, *Pillsbury Plus* (¹/₁₂ package)	180	34.0	4.0	NA	NA	275
●★ Bundt, fudge, cake/filling/glaze, *Pillsbury* (¹/₁₂ package)	260	49.0	6.0	NA	NA	405
●★ Bundt, lemon, cake/filling/glaze, *Pillsbury* (¹/₁₂ package)	290	59.0	5.0	NA	NA	375
●★ Bundt, marble, cake/filling/glaze, *Pillsbury* (¹/₁₂ package)	280	51.0	7.0	NA	NA	310
●★ Butter flavor cake/streusel/glaze, *Pillsbury Streusel Swirl* (¹/₁₆ package)	200	38.0	5.0	NA	NA	220
●★ Butter yellow, *Betty Crocker Super Moist* (¹/₁₂ package)	180	36.0	3.0	NA	NA	240
★■ Cake and cookie, prepared, *Featherweight* (1″ slice)	170	24.0	7.0	NA	NA	5
●★ Carrot, *Betty Crocker Super Moist* (¹/₁₂ package)	180	34.0	4.0	NA	NA	240
●★ Chocolate/chocolate frosting, *Betty Crocker Stir 'N Frost* (¹/₆ package)	210	38.0	6.0	NA	NA	240
●★ Chocolate, *Duncan Hines Deluxe II* (¹/₁₂ package)	190	33.0	5.0	1.8	NA	390
●★ Chocolate, *Duncan Hines Pudding Recipe* (¹/₁₂ package)	180	34.0	4.0	NA	NA	405
★ Chocolate flavor, sugar restricted, prepared, *Sweet 'N Low* (¹/₁₀ cake)	90	16.0	2.0	NA	5	20
●★ Chocolate fudge, prepared, *General Mills Light Style* (¹/₁₂ cake)	160	30.0	3.0	NA	NA	NA
●★ Chocolate, *Pillsbury* (¹/₁₂ package)	180	32.0	5.0	NA	NA	355

Alerts: ● Sodium ★ Sugar ■ Cholesterol

Food Description	Calories	Carbohydrates (grams)	Fat (grams)	Saturated Fat (grams)	Cholesterol (milligrams)	Sodium (milligrams)
●★Cinnamon, cake/streusel/glaze, *Pillsbury Streusel Swirl* (¹/₁₂ package)	280	51.0	7.0	NA	NA	250
●★Coconut pecan, *Betty Crocker Snackin' Cake* (¹/₉ package)	190	30.0	7.0	NA	NA	245
●★Devil's food, prepared, *General Mills Light Style* (¹/₁₂ cake)	160	29.0	3.0	NA	NA	NA
●★Fudge, *Duncan Hines Butter Recipe* (¹/₁₂ package)	190	34.0	4.0	2.5	NA	240
●★Fudge marble, *Duncan Hines Deluxe II* (¹/₁₂ package)	190	34.0	5.0	NA	NA	240
●★German chocolate, *Pillsbury Plus* (¹/₁₂ package)	180	34.0	4.0	NA	NA	325
●★Gingerbread, *Betty Crocker* (¹/₉ package)	200	36.0	5.0	NA	NA	315
●★Gingerbread, prepared (2¾" square piece)	174	32.2	4.3	1.1	1	191
●★Golden chocolate chip, *Betty Crocker Snackin' Cake* (¹/₉ package)	190	34.0	5.0	NA	NA	245
Lemon, dietetic, *Batter-Lite* (¹/₁₀ package)	100	15.0	3.0	2.0	Tr.	16
●★Lemon/lemon frosting, *Betty Crocker Stir 'N Frost* (¹/₆ package)	220	41.0	5.0	NA	NA	240
●★Lemon, prepared, *General Mills Light Style* (¹/₁₂ cake)	160	29.0	3.0	NA	NA	NA
●★Lemon pudding, *Betty Crocker* (¹/₆ package)	220	45.0	4.0	NA	NA	260
★Low sodium, prepared, *Featherweight* (½" slice)	200	20.0	12.0	NA	NA	6
●★Orange, *Duncan Hines Deluxe II* (¹/₁₂ package)	190	34.0	5.0	NA	NA	240
●★Pound, *Betty Crocker* (¹/₁₂ package)	180	27.0	7.0	NA	NA	140
●★Quick bread, apricot nut, *Pillsbury* (¹/₁₂ package)	150	27.0	4.0	NA	NA	145
●★Quick bread, brown, with raisins, *B & M* (1.6 oz. slice)	80	18.0	NA	NA	NA	220
●★Quick bread, cranberry, *Pillsbury* (¹/₁₂ package)	150	28.0	3.0	NA	NA	145
●★Quick bread, date, *Pillsbury* (¹/₁₆ package)	120	25.0	2.0	NA	NA	120
●★Quick bread, oatmeal raisin, *Pillsbury* (¹/₁₆ package)	110	22.0	2.0	NA	NA	100

Alerts: ● Sodium ★ Sugar ■ Cholesterol

Food Description	Calories	Carbohydrates (grams)	Fat (grams)	Saturated Fat (grams)	Cholesterol (milligrams)	Sodium (milligrams)
●★Raisin, *Betty Crocker Snackin' Cake* (¹/₉ package)	180	33.0	4.0	NA	NA	250
●★Sour cream white, *Betty Crocker Super Moist* (¹/₁₂ package)	180	36.0	3.0	NA	NA	245
●★Strawberry flavor, *Pillsbury Plus* (¹/₁₂ package)	180	34.0	4.0	NA	NA	280
●★Vanilla, *Duncan Hines Pudding Recipe* (¹/₁₂ package)	180	36.0	3.0	NA	NA	280
●White, dietetic, *Batter-Lite* (¹/₁₀ package)	100	15.0	4.0	2.0	Tr.	95
●★White, *Duncan Hines Deluxe II* (¹/₁₂ package)	190	34.0	5.0	NA	NA	230
★White, sugar restricted, prepared, *Sweet 'N Low* (¹/₁₀ cake)	90	16.0	2.0	NA	5	20
●★Yellow, *Pillsbury* (¹/₁₂ package)	180	33.0	5.0	NA	NA	275
●★Yellow, prepared, *General Mills Light Style* (¹/₁₂ cake)	160	29.0	3.0	NA	NA	NA
ICINGS						
●★Cherry, *Betty Crocker Creamy Deluxe* (¹/₁₂ can)	170	28.0	6.0	NA	NA	95
●★Chocolate, *Betty Crocker Light Style* (¹/₁₂ package)	100	18.0	3.0	NA	NA	55
●★Chocolate flavored, *Betty Crocker Creamy Deluxe* (¹/₁₂ can)	170	25.0	8.0	NA	NA	95
●★Chocolate flavor, prepared, *Sweet 'N Low* (1½ tsp.)	30	3.0	2.0	NA	5	10
●★Chocolate fudge flavor, *Pillsbury Frosting Supreme* (¹/₁₂ can)	160	24.0	7.0	NA	NA	90
●★■Chocolate, homemade (1 cup)	1034	185.4	38.2	21.3	44	167
●★Coconut, homemade (1 cup)	604	124.3	12.8	11.0	0	195
●★Cream cheese flavor, *Pillsbury Frosting Supreme* (¹/₁₂ can)	164	27.0	6.0	NA	NA	80
●★Dark chocolate fudge, prepared, *Betty Crocker* (¹/₁₂ package)	170	30.0	6.0	NA	NA	100
●★Lemon, *Betty Crocker Light Style* (¹/₁₂ package)	100	19.0	3.0	NA	NA	50
●★Milk chocolate flavor, *Pillsbury Frosting Supreme* (¹/₁₂ can)	160	25.0	6.0	NA	NA	50

Alerts: ● Sodium   ★ Sugar   ■ Cholesterol

Food Description	Calories	Carbohydrates (grams)	Fat (grams)	Saturated Fat (grams)	Cholesterol (milligrams)	Sodium (milligrams)
●★Strawberry flavor, *Pillsbury Frosting Supreme* (¹/₁₂ can)	160	27.0	6.0	NA	NA	45
●★Vanilla, *Betty Crocker Light Style* (¹/₁₂ package)	100	19.0	3.0	NA	NA	50
●★Vanilla flavor, *Pillsbury Frosting Supreme* (¹/₁₂ can)	160	27.0	6.0	NA	NA	80
●★White, fluffy, *Betty Crocker* (¹/₁₂ package)	60	16.0	0	0	NA	40
●★■White, homemade (1 cup)	1199	260.3	21.1	11.6	64	156
●★White, prepared, *Sweet 'N Low* (1½ tsp.)	30	3.0	2.0	NA	5	10
●★White sour cream, *Betty Crocker Creamy Deluxe* (¹/₁₂ can)	160	27.0	6.0	NA	NA	95

Candy

Food Description	Calories	Carbohydrates (grams)	Fat (grams)	Saturated Fat (grams)	Cholesterol (milligrams)	Sodium (milligrams)
Bars						
●★*Baby Ruth* (1.8 oz.)	260	31.0	11.0	8.0	0	100
●★*Butterfinger* (1.6 oz.)	220	28.0	10.0	8.0	0	70
★Chocolate, special dark, *Hershey* (1.05 oz.)	160	19.0	9.0	NA	NA	NA
●★*Crunch* (1 oz.)	150	18.0	8.0	NA	5	55
★*Golden Almond* (1 oz.)	160	12.0	11.0	NA	NA	20
★*$100,000* (1 oz.)	140	20.0	6.0	NA	NA	50
★*Kit Kat* (1.12 oz.)	160	19.0	8.0	NA	NA	30
★*Krackel* (1.2 oz.)	180	20.0	10.0	NA	NA	50
★*Mars* (1.52 oz.)	210	27.0	10.0	NA	NA	NA
★Milk chocolate, *Hershey* (1.05 oz.)	160	17.0	10.0	NA	NA	30
★Milk chocolate, *Nestle* (1 oz.)	150	17.0	8.0	NA	5	25
★Milk chocolate, with almonds, *Hershey* (1.05 oz.)	160	16.0	10.0	NA	NA	25
★Milk chocolate, with almonds, *Nestle* (1 oz.)	150	17.0	9.0	NA	5	20
★*Milky Way* (1.9 oz.)	240	40.0	8.0	NA	NA	NA
★*Mr. Goodbar* (1.3 oz.)	200	18.0	12.0	NA	NA	20
★Peanut (1 oz.)	146	13.4	9.1	2.0	0	2

Alerts: ● Sodium ★ Sugar ■ Cholesterol

Food Description	Calories	Carbohydrates (grams)	Fat (grams)	Saturated Fat (grams)	Cholesterol (milligrams)	Sodium (milligrams)
★Peanut Crunch, Sahadi (0.75 oz.)	110	6.0	7.0	NA	NA	NA
★Reggie (2 oz.)	290	29.0	17.0	NA	0	40
★Rice Crisp, Featherweight (2 sections)	100	9.0	6.0	NA	NA	NA
★Snickers (1.8 oz.)	250	30.0	12.0	NA	NA	NA
★Summit (0.61 oz.)	97	9.0	6.0	NA	NA	NA
★3 Musketeers (2.05 oz.)	250	44.0	8.0	NA	NA	NA
★Twix (0.86 oz.)	121	14.0	5.0	NA	NA	NA
●★Whatchamacallit (1.15 oz.)	170	18.0	10.0	NA	NA	70
★Butterscotch (1 oz.)	113	26.9	1.0	0.5	3	18
●★Candy corn (1 cup)	728	179.2	4.0	1.0	0	424
★Caramel creams, Gaetze's (3 oz.)	323	67.6	3.9	NA	NA	NA
●★Caramel Nip, Pearson (1.75 oz.)	220	43.0	5.0	1.0	0	130
●★Caramels (1 oz.)	113	21.7	2.9	1.6	1	64
●★Caramel, with nuts (1 oz.)	121	20.0	4.6	1.6	1	57
★Chocolate, Hershey Kisses (6 pieces)	150	16.0	9.0	NA	NA	25
★Chocolate Parfait, Pearson (1.75 oz.)	240	40.0	8.0	1.0	0	20
●★Coffee Nip, Pearson (1.75 oz.)	220	43.0	5.0	1.0	0	130
★Coffioca, Pearson (1.75 oz.)	240	40.0	8.0	1.0	0	20
★Fructose tablet, carob flavor, Batter-Lite (0.07 oz.)	8	2.0	0	0	0	NA
★Fructose tablet, cherry flavor, Batter-Lite (0.07 oz.)	8	2.0	0	0	0	NA
★Fruit chews, Starburst (1 oz.)	110	24.0	2.0	NA	NA	NA
★Fudge, chocolate (1 oz.)	113	21.3	3.5	1.2	1	53
●★Fudge, vanilla (1 oz.)	113	21.2	3.1	0.8	1	59
★Gum drops (1 oz.)	98	24.8	0.2	0	0	9
★Gum drops, low calorie, assorted flavors, Sug'r Like (1 drop)	3	1.0	0	0	0	1
★Hard, assorted flavors, Featherweight (1 piece)	12	3.0	0	0	0	NA
★Hard, dietetic, assorted flavors, Sug'r Like (1 piece)	12	3.0	0	0	0	NA
★Jelly beans (1 oz.)	104	26.4	0.1	0	0	3
●★Licorice Nip, Pearson (1.75 oz.)	220	43.0	5.0	1.0	0	130
★M&M's, peanut (1.51 oz.)	220	25.0	11.0	NA	NA	NA
★M&M's, plain (1.44 oz.)	200	28.0	9.0	NA	NA	NA
★Marshmallow (1 large)	23	5.8	0	0	0	2

Alerts: ● Sodium ★ Sugar ■ Cholesterol

Food Description	Calories	Carbohydrates (grams)	Fat (grams)	Saturated Fat (grams)	Cholesterol (milligrams)	Sodium (milligrams)
★Milk chocolate (1 oz.)	147	16.1	9.2	5.1	6	26
★Milk chocolate, with almonds (1 oz.)	151	14.5	10.1	4.5	5	22
★Milk chocolate, with peanuts (1 oz.)	154	12.6	10.8	4.5	4	18
★*Mint Parfait, Pearson* (1.75 oz.)	240	40.0	8.0	1.0	0	20
★Mints, chocolate, *Royals* (1.26 oz.)	182	25.0	8.0	NA	0	NA
★Mints, *Pep-O-Mint, Life Savers* (1 mint)	7	2.0	0	0	0	NA
Mints, spearmint, *Featherweight* (1 mint)	4	1.0	0.5	Tr.	0	NA
Mints, sugarless, peppermint, *Sug'r Like* (1 mint)	4	1.0	0.5	Tr.	0	NA
★Mints, *Tic Tac,* all flavors (1 mint)	2	0.4	0	0	0	0
★Mints, wintermint, *Featherweight* (1 mint)	4	1.0	0.5	Tr.	0	NA
●★Peanut butter cup, *Reese's* (1.2 oz.)	180	17.0	11.0	NA	NA	110
●★*Peanut Crunch, Sahadi* (20 pieces)	170	10.0	11.0	NA	NA	NA
●★Peanut, *Old Fashioned, Planters* (1 oz.)	140	15.0	15.0	3.0	0	120
●★Peanuts, chocolate-coated (1 cup)	954	66.5	70.2	18.3	2	102
●★Raisins, chocolate-coated (1 cup)	808	134.0	32.5	18.1	19	121
●★*Rolo* (1 oz.)	140	19.0	6.0	NA	NA	65

Cereals

COLD, READY-TO-EAT CEREALS						
●★*All-Bran* (1 oz.)	70	21.0	0	0	0	160
●★*Alpha-Bits* (1 cup)	110	24.0	1.0	0	0	195
●★*Body Buddies,* brown sugar and honey (1 oz.)	110	25.0	1.0	0	0	230

Alerts: ● Sodium ★ Sugar ■ Cholesterol

Food Description	Calories	Carbohydrates (grams)	Fat (grams)	Saturated Fat (grams)	Cholesterol (milligrams)	Sodium (milligrams)
•★Bran Chex (⅔ cup)	110	20.0	1.0	0	0	300
•★Buc Wheats (¾ cup)	110	23.0	1.0	0	0	270
•★Cap'N Crunch (1 oz.)	110	24.0	2.0	1.0	0	193
•★Cheerios (1 oz.)	110	20.0	2.0	0	0	330
•★Cheerios, Honey Nut (¾ cup)	110	23.0	1.0	0	0	255
•★Cocoa Krispies (1 oz.)	110	25.0	0	0	0	215
•★Cocoa Pebbles (⅞ cup)	110	25.0	2.0	NA	0	165
•★Cocoa Puffs (1 cup)	110	25.0	1.0	0	0	205
•★Corn Bran (⅔ cup)	110	24.0	1.0	0	0	NA
•★Corn Chex (1 cup)	110	25.0	0	0	0	325
•★Corn flake crumbs (1 cup)	328	72.5	0.3	0	0	854
★Corn flakes, low sodium, Featherweight (1¼ cup)	110	25.0	0	0	0	10
•★Country Corn Flakes (1 oz.)	110	25.0	1.0	0	0	310
•★Cracklin' Bran (1 oz.)	120	20.0	4.0	NA	0	160
•★Crispy Wheats 'n Raisins (¾ cup)	110	23.0	1.0	0	0	185
★C. W. Post (1 oz.)	130	20.0	4.0	NA	0	55
★C. W. Post, with raisins (1 oz.)	120	21.0	4.0	NA	0	50
•★Fortified Oat Flakes, Post (1 oz.)	100	20.0	1.0	0	0	275
•★40% Bran Flakes, Kellogg's (1 oz.)	90	22.0	1.0	0	0	265
•★40% Bran Flakes, Post (⅔ cup)	90	23.0	1.0	0	0	225
•★Froot Loops (1 oz.)	110	25.0	0	0	0	130
★Frosted Mini-Wheats (1 oz.)	110	23.0	0	0	0	10
•★Fruity Pebbles (⅞ cup)	110	25.0	2.0	NA	0	160
•★Golden Grahams (1 oz.)	110	24.0	1.0	0	0	345
•★Grape Nuts (1 oz.)	100	23.0	1.0	0	0	195
•★Heartland (1 oz.)	120	18.0	4.0	NA	0	NA
•★Heartland, with coconut (1 oz.)	130	18.0	5.0	NA	0	NA
•★Heartland, with raisins (1 oz.)	120	18.0	4.0	NA	0	NA
•★Honey Bran (⅞ cup)	100	20.0	1.0	0	0	200
•★Honey-Comb (1 oz.)	110	25.0	1.0	0	0	195
•★King Vitaman (¾ cup)	120	23.3	2.4	NA	0	215
•★Kix (1½ cups)	110	24.0	1.0	0	0	315
•★Life (⅔ cup)	110	19.0	1.0	0	0	NA
•★Life, cinnamon flavored (⅔ cup)	110	19.0	1.0	0	0	NA
•★Lucky Charms (1 oz.)	110	24.0	1.0	0	0	185
•★Most (1 oz.)	110	22.0	0	0	0	150
★Nature Valley, cinnamon-raisin (1 oz.)	130	19.0	5.0	NA	0	45

Alerts: • Sodium ★ Sugar ■ Cholesterol

Food Description	Calories	Carbohydrates (grams)	Fat (grams)	Saturated Fat (grams)	Cholesterol (milligrams)	Sodium (milligrams)
★Nature Valley Granola, coconut and honey (1 oz.)	150	18.0	7.0	NA	0	55
★Nature Valley Granola, fruit and nut (1 oz.)	130	20.0	4.0	NA	0	50
★Nature Valley Granola, toasted oats (1 oz.)	130	19.0	5.0	NA	0	50
●★100% Bran, Nabisco (½ cup)	70	21.0	2.0	0	0	NA
★100% Natural, Quaker (¼ cup)	140	17.0	6.0	NA	Tr.	18
★100% Natural, with raisins and dates, Quaker (¼ cup)	130	18.0	5.0	NA	Tr.	NA
●★Post Toasties (1 oz.)	110	24.0	1.0	0	0	305
●★Product 19 (¾ cup)	110	24.0	0	0	0	175
Puffed Rice, Malt-O-Meal (½ oz.)	50	12.0	0	0	0	10
Puffed Rice, Quaker (1 cup)	50	13.0	0	0	0	10
Puffed Wheat, Malt-O-Meal (½ oz.)	50	11.0	0	0	0	10
Puffed Wheat, Quaker (1 cup)	54	10.8	0.2	0	0	1
●★Quisp (¾ cup)	120	23.0	2.0	NA	0	NA
●★Raisin Bran, Kellogg's (1 oz.)	90	22.0	1.0	0	0	170
●★Raisins, Rice, and Rye, Kellogg's (1 cup)	140	31.0	0	0	0	280
●★Rice Chex (1 cup)	110	25.0	0	0	0	275
★Rice, crisp, Featherweight (1 oz.)	110	25.0	0	0	0	10
●★Rice Krinkles (1 oz.)	110	26.0	1.0	0	0	185
●★Rice Krispies (1 oz.)	110	25.0	0	0	0	340
★Shredded Wheat, Quaker (2 biscuits)	104	22.0	0.4	0	0	2
★Shredded Wheat, spoon size, Nabisco (⅔ cup)	110	23.0	1.0	0	0	10
●★Special K (1 oz.)	110	21.0	0	0	0	265
●★Sugar Frosted Flakes (1 oz.)	110	26.0	0	0	0	230
●★Sugar Smacks (1 oz.)	110	25.0	0	0	0	75
★Super Sugar Crisp (⅞ cup)	110	26.0	1.0	0	0	35
●★Team (1 cup)	110	24.0	1.0	0	0	NA
●★Toasty O's (1 oz.)	110	20.0	2.0	NA	0	280
●★Total, corn (1 oz.)	110	24.0	1.0	0	0	310
●★Total, whole wheat (1 cup)	110	23.0	1.0	0	0	375
●★Trix (1 oz.)	110	25.0	1.0	0	0	170
●★Waffelos (1 cup)	110	24.0	1.0	0	0	150
●★Wheat and Raisin Chex (¾ cup)	120	30.0	0	0	0	250
●★Wheat Chex (1 oz.)	110	23.0	1.0	0	0	240
Wheat germ, Kretschmer (¼ cup)	110	13.0	3.0	0.6	0	1

Alerts: ● Sodium ★ Sugar ■ Cholesterol

Food Description	Calories	Carbohydrates (grams)	Fat (grams)	Saturated Fat (grams)	Cholesterol (milligrams)	Sodium (milligrams)
★Wheat germ, with brown sugar and honey, *Kretschmer* (1 oz.)	110	17.0	2.0	0	0	31
●★*Wheaties* (¾ cup)	110	23.0	1.0	0	0	370
HOT CEREALS						
★*Coco-Wheats* (3 Tbsp.)	130	28.0	1.0	0.2	0	3
Cream of Wheat (1 oz.)	100	22.0	0	0	0	10
Cream of Wheat, instant (1 oz.)	100	22.0	0	0	0	4
●★*Cream of Wheat, Mix 'n Eat* (1 oz. packet)	100	21.0	0	0	0	265
●★*Cream of Wheat, Mix 'n Eat*, baked apple with cinnamon (1¼ oz. packet)	130	29.0	0	0	0	275
●★*Cream of Wheat, Mix 'n Eat*, maple and brown sugar (1¼ oz. packet)	130	29.0	0	0	0	NA
●*Cream of Wheat*, quick (1 oz.)	100	22.0	0	0	0	130
Farina, *Hot 'n Creamy, Quaker* (⅙ cup)	101	21.7	0.2	0	0	1
Farina, *Pillsbury* (¾ oz.)	80	17.0	0	0	0	0
★Hominy grits, white, instant, *Quaker* (0.8 oz. packet)	80	18.0	0	0	0	0
★*Maltex* (1 oz.)	117	21.0	1.0	0	0	3
Malt-O-Meal (1 oz.)	100	22.0	0	0	0	2
●★Oatmeal, instant, apples and cinnamon, *Quaker* (1¼ oz. packet)	130	26.0	2.0	0.3	0	181
●★Oatmeal, instant, bran and spice, *H-O* (1 packet)	170	33.1	1.8	Tr.	0	305
●★Oatmeal, instant, cinnamon and spice, *Quaker* (1⅝ oz. packet)	170	34.0	2.0	0	0	NA
●★Oatmeal, instant, maple and brown sugar, *Quaker* (1½ oz. packet)	160	31.0	2.0	0	0	227
★Oatmeal, instant, maple flavored, *Maypo* (¼ cup)	123	19.0	1.0	0	0	2
●Oatmeal, instant, *Quaker* (1 oz. packet)	100	17.0	2.0	0.4	0	252
●★Oatmeal, instant, raisins and spice, *Quaker* (1½ oz. packet)	160	31.0	2.0	0.4	0	227
★Oats, *Maypo Vermont Style* (1 oz.)	122	20.0	1.0	0	0	4

Alerts: ● Sodium ★ Sugar ■ Cholesterol

Food Description	Calories	Carbohydrates (grams)	Fat (grams)	Saturated Fat (grams)	Cholesterol (milligrams)	Sodium (milligrams)
Oats, *Old Fashioned, Quaker* (⅓ cup)	110	18.0	2.0	0.4	0	1
Oats, quick, *H-O* (½ cup)	130	23.0	2.0	Tr.	0	5
Oats, quick, *Quaker* (⅓ cup)	110	18.0	2.0	0.4	0	1
Oats, *3 Minute* (1 oz.)	110	18.0	2.0	Tr.	0	10
Ralston (1 oz.)	90	20.0	1.0	0	0	5
Wheatena (1 oz.)	120	21.0	1.0	0	0	2
Whole wheat, natural, *Quaker* (⅓ cup)	100	20.0	1.0	0.1	0	10

Cheese and Eggs

NATURAL CHEESE

Food Description	Calories	Carbohydrates (grams)	Fat (grams)	Saturated Fat (grams)	Cholesterol (milligrams)	Sodium (milligrams)
●■ Blarney, *Otto Roth* (1 oz.)	103	0.4	8.1	NA	25	300
●■ Blue (1 oz.)	104	0.6	8.6	4.8	25	199
●■ Blue, *Land O' Lakes* (1 oz.)	100	1.0	8.0	5.0	21	396
●■ Blue, *Stella* (1 oz.)	100	1.0	8.0	NA	21	NA
●■ Brick (1 oz.)	105	0.5	8.6	4.8	26	199
●■ Brick, *Land O' Lakes* (1 oz.)	110	1.0	8.0	5.0	27	159
●■ Brick, *Otto Roth* (1 oz.)	105	1.0	8.0	NA	27	159
●■ Brie (1 oz.)	95	0.1	7.9	NA	28	178
●■ Brie, *Otto Roth* (1 oz.)	85	0.1	7.3	NA	19	200
●■ Camembert (1 oz.)	85	0.5	7.0	3.9	26	199
●■ Cheddar, domestic (1 oz.)	113	0.6	9.1	5.0	28	199
●■ Cheddar, goat's milk, *Clayton* (1 oz.)	110	1.0	9.0	NA	14	NA
●■ Cheddar, *Land O' Lakes* (1 oz.)	110	1.0	9.0	6.0	30	176
●■ Cheddar, *Otto Roth* (1 oz.)	114	1.0	9.0	NA	30	176
■ Cheddar, unsalted, *Featherweight* (1 oz.)	110	0	9.0	NA	NA	5
●■ Cheshire (1 oz.)	110	1.4	8.9	NA	29	198
●■ Colby (1 oz.)	112	0.7	9.1	5.7	27	171
●■ Colby, *Land O' Lakes* (1 oz.)	100	1.0	9.0	6.0	27	171
■ Colby, low sodium, *Pauly* (1 oz.)	110	1.0	10.0	NA	NA	5
●■ Colby, *Stella* (1 oz.)	110	1.0	9.0	NA	27	NA
■ Colby, unsalted, *Featherweight* (1 oz.)	110	0	9.0	NA	NA	5

Alerts: ● Sodium ★ Sugar ■ Cholesterol

Food Description	Calories	Carbohydrates (grams)	Fat (grams)	Saturated Fat (grams)	Cholesterol (milligrams)	Sodium (milligrams)
• Cottage, creamed, 1% fat (½ cup)	82	3.1	1.2	0.7	5	459
• Cottage, creamed, 2% fat (½ cup)	101	4.1	2.2	1.4	9	459
• Cottage, creamed, 4.2% fat (1 oz.)	30	0.8	1.2	0.7	5	114
• Cottage, dry curd, 0.3% fat (1 oz.)	24	0.8	0.1	0	2	82
•■ Edam (1 oz.)	101	0.4	7.9	5.0	25	274
•■ Edam, *Stella* (1 oz.)	100	1.0	8.0	NA	25	NA
•■ Farmers, *Otto Roth* (1 oz.)	110	0.3	7.9	NA	NA	170
•■ Feta (1 oz.)	75	1.2	6.0	4.2	25	316
•■ Fontina (1 oz.)	110	0.4	8.8	5.4	33	NA
•■ Fontinella, *Stella* (1 oz.)	120	1.0	10.0	NA	33	NA
•■ Gorgonzola, *Stella* (1 oz.)	100	1.0	8.0	NA	21	NA
•■ Gouda (1 oz.)	101	0.6	7.8	5.0	32	232
■ Gouda, Holland, no salt added, *Otto Roth* (1 oz.)	100	1.0	8.0	NA	NA	10
•■ Gouda, *Land O' Lakes* (1 oz.)	100	1.0	8.0	5.0	32	232
■ Gouda, low sodium, *Otto Roth* (1 oz.)	90	NA	8.5	NA	25	7
•■ Gouda, *Stella* (1 oz.)	100	1.0	8.0	NA	32	NA
•■ Gruyere (1 oz.)	117	0.1	9.2	5.4	31	95
•■ Gruyere, *Swiss Knight* (1 oz.)	100	1.0	8.0	NA	25	360
•■ La Vacke, *Otto Roth* (1 oz.)	72	0.7	6.0	NA	18	312
• La Vacke, reduced calorie, *Otto Roth* (¾ oz.)	35	1.0	2.0	NA	6	234
•■ Limburger (1 oz.)	98	0.6	7.9	4.4	28	201
•■ Monterey (1 oz.)	106	0.2	8.6	NA	NA	152
•■ Monterey Jack, *Land O' Lakes* (1 oz.)	100	1.0	8.0	NA	27	152
• Mozzarella, *Land O' Lakes* (1 oz.)	80	1.0	5.0	3.0	15	150
• Mozzarella, part skim, low moisture, *Kraft* (1 oz.)	80	1.0	5.0	3.0	15	220
•■ Muenster (1 oz.)	104	0.3	8.5	5.4	27	178
•■ Muenster, *Land O' Lakes* (1 oz.)	100	1.0	9.0	5.0	27	178
•■ Muenster, *Otto Roth* (1 oz.)	107	1.0	8.0	NA	26	74
•■ Parmesan, grated (1 Tbsp.)	23	0.2	1.5	1.0	4	93
•■ Parmesan, hard (1 oz.)	111	0.9	7.3	4.6	19	454
Premonde, *Otto Roth* (1 oz.)	102	0.4	8.0	NA	2	3
•■ Provolone (1 oz.)	100	0.6	7.6	4.8	20	248
•■ Provolone, *Land O' Lakes* (1 oz.)	90	1.0	7.0	5.0	20	248
•■ Provolone, *Stella* (1 oz.)	90	1.0	7.0	NA	19	NA

Alerts: • Sodium ★ Sugar ■ Cholesterol

Food Description	Calories	Carbohydrates (grams)	Fat (grams)	Saturated Fat (grams)	Cholesterol (milligrams)	Sodium (milligrams)
●■ Romano (1 oz.)	110	1.0	7.6	NA	29	340
●■ Romano, *Stella* (1 oz.)	100	1.0	7.0	NA	29	NA
●■ Roquefort (1 oz.)	104	0.6	8.6	4.8	25	199
● Scandic, *Otto Roth* (1 oz.)	110	0.3	9.0	NA	1	218
●■ Semisoft, skim milk, colored or white, *Weight Watchers* (1 oz.)	80	1.0	5.0	NA	NA	190
● Skim milk, white or yellow, *Somerset* (1 oz.)	70	1.0	4.0	NA	13	170
● Swedish, low cholesterol, *Skandic* (1 oz.)	110	NA	9.0	NA	1	220
●■ Swiss, *Land O' Lakes* (1 oz.)	110	0	8.0	5.0	26	74
■ Swiss, no salt added, *Dorman* (1 oz.)	105	1.0	8.0	NA	NA	10
● Tivoli Danalette, *Otto Roth* (1 oz.)	62	0.3	2.8	1.7	8	198
PROCESSED CHEESE AND SPREADS						
● American, *Borden Lite-Line* (1 oz.)	50	1.0	2.0	NA	10	NA
●■ American, *Dorman* (1 oz.)	90	2.0	7.0	5.6	27	406
● American, imitation, low calorie, *Unique* (1 oz.)	80	1.0	6.0	NA	5	385
●■ American, *Kraft* (1 oz.)	90	2.0	7.0	4.0	20	405
●■ American, *Kraft Velveeta* (1 oz.)	80	2.0	6.0	3.0	20	430
●■ American, *Land O' Lakes* (1 oz.)	110	1.0	9.0	6.0	27	384
●■ American, *Otto Roth* (1 oz.)	106	1.0	9.0	NA	25	406
● American, skim, *Borden* (1 oz.)	70	1.0	5.0	NA	10	NA
● American, skim, *Weight Watchers* (1 oz.)	50	1.0	2.0	NA	8	530
●■ American, spread (1 oz.)	78	2.2	5.8	3.2	17	439
●■ American, spread, *Snack Mate* (1 oz.)	80	2.0	6.0	NA	NA	NA
●■ American Swiss, *Land O' Lakes* (1 oz.)	110	1.0	9.0	5.0	20	303
●■ Blue cheese food, *Wispride* (1 oz.)	100	2.0	7.0	NA	NA	265
●■ Caraway cheese food, *Land O' Lakes* (1 oz.)	90	2.0	7.0	4.0	20	318
●■ Cheddar cheese food, sharp, cold pack, *Land O' Lakes* (1 oz.)	90	2.0	7.0	4.0	18	274

Alerts: ● Sodium ★ Sugar ■ Cholesterol

Food Description	Calories	Carbohydrates (grams)	Fat (grams)	Saturated Fat (grams)	Cholesterol (milligrams)	Sodium (milligrams)
●■Cheddar, spread, *Snack Mate* (1 oz.)	80	2.0	6.0	NA	NA	NA
●■Cream, *Philadelphia* (1 oz.)	100	1.0	10.0	5.0	25	110
●■*Golden Velvet,* spread, *Land O' Lakes* (1 oz.)	80	2.0	6.0	4.0	16	381
●Mozzarella, imitation, low calorie, *Uni-Chef* (1 oz.)	90	1.0	6.0	NA	7	360
●■Neufchatel (1 oz.)	74	0.8	6.6	4.2	22	113
●■Neufchatel, low fat, *Kraft* (1 oz.)	80	1.0	7.0	5.0	20	110
●■Onion flavor cheese food, *Land O' Lakes* (1 oz.)	90	2.0	7.0	4.0	18	325
●Semi-soft, imitation, *Dorman's Lo-Chol* (1 oz.)	105	0	9.0	1.8	4	130
●■Swiss (1 oz.)	95	0.6	7.1	4.6	24	388
●■Swiss cheese food, *Wispride* (1 oz.)	100	7.0	7.0	NA	NA	195
EGGS						
■Duck, raw (1 egg)	134	0.5	10.2	3.5	355	86
●■Fried (1 large egg)	99	0.1	7.9	2.9	257	156
●■Goose, raw (1 egg)	266	1.9	19.1	7.2	723	175
■Hardboiled (1 large egg)	82	0.5	5.8	1.9	253	61
●■Omelet, prepared with butter/milk (1 large egg)	95	1.4	7.1	2.8	248	155
●■Omelette, Spanish style, frozen, *Campbell's* (8 oz.)	250	14.0	18.0	NA	NA	783
●■Omelette, with cheese and ham, frozen, *Campbell's* (8 oz.)	380	13.0	28.0	NA	NA	1402
●■Poached (1 large egg)	82	0.4	5.8	1.9	252	136
■Raw (1 large egg)	82	0.5	5.8	1.9	253	61
●■Scrambled (1 large egg)	111	1.5	8.3	2.8	260	165
●Substitute, *Egg Supreme* (¼ cup)	40	2.0	0	0	0	112
●Substitute, no cholesterol, *Egg Beaters* (¼ cup)	40	0.3	0	0	0	130
■Turkey, raw (1 egg)	135	1.3	9.3	3.2	399	97
White, raw (1 large)	19	0.3	0	0	0	56
■Yolk, raw (1 large)	59	0.1	5.2	1.7	252	9

Alerts: ● Sodium ★ Sugar ■ Cholesterol

Condiments and Baking Products

Food Description	Calories	Carbohydrates (grams)	Fat (grams)	Saturated Fat (grams)	Cholesterol (milligrams)	Sodium (milligrams)
BAKING PRODUCTS						
Baking powder, low sodium, (1 tsp.)	7	1.8	0	0	0	0
Baking powder, low sodium, *Featherweight* (1 tsp.)	8	2.0	0	0	0	2
• Baking powder, sodium aluminum sulfate, with monocalcium phosphate monohydrate and calcium carbonate (1 tsp.)	2	0.6	0	0	0	348
• Baking powder, sodium aluminum sulfate, with monocalcium phosphate monohydrate and calcium sulfate (1 tsp.)	3	0.7	0	0	0	290
• Baking soda (1 tsp.)	0	0	0	0	0	952
★ Butterscotch flavor morsels, *Nestle* (1 oz.)	150	19.0	7.0	NA	0	20
★ Cherries, candied (¾ cup)	383	98.0	0.2	0	0	2
Chocolate						
Bitter, grated (1 oz.)	143	8.2	15.0	8.4	0	1
★ Bittersweet (1 oz.)	135	13.3	11.3	6.3	0	1
★ *Choco-Bake* (1 oz.)	170	12.0	14.0	NA	0	10
★ Flavored morsels, *Baker* (1 oz.)	130	20.0	7.0	NA	0	4
★ *Hershey* (1 oz.)	190	7.0	16.0	NA	0	NA
★ Milk, morsels, *Nestle* (1 oz.)	150	17.0	9.0	NA	5	25
★ Semi-sweet, *Baker* (1 oz.)	130	17.0	9.0	NA	0	1
★ Semi-sweet, bits, *Nestle* (1 oz.)	150	18.0	8.0	NA	0	10
★ Semi-sweet, chips, *Hershey* (¼ cup)	220	26.0	12.0	NA	0	NA
★ Sweet, German, *Baker* (1 oz.)	140	17.0	9.0	NA	0	Tr.
Unsweetened, *Baker* (1 oz.)	140	9.0	14.0	NA	0	4
•★ Citron, candied (1 oz.)	89	22.7	0.1	0	0	82
•★ Coconut, shredded, *Baker Premium* (¼ cup)	100	9.0	7.0	NA	0	50

Alerts: • Sodium ★ Sugar ■ Cholesterol

Food Description	Calories	Carbohydrates (grams)	Fat (grams)	Saturated Fat (grams)	Cholesterol (milligrams)	Sodium (milligrams)
★Ginger root, candied (1 oz.)	96	24.7	0.1	0	0	17
★Grapefruit peel, candied (1 oz.)	90	22.9	0.1	0	0	0
★Lemon peel, candied (1 oz.)	90	22.9	0.1	0	0	0
Lemon peel, grated (1 tsp.)	1	0.3	0	0	0	0
Malt, dry (1 oz.)	104	21.9	0.5	0	0	22
★Orange peel, candied (1 oz.)	90	22.9	0.1	0	0	0
Orange peel, grated (1 tsp.)	2.0	0.5	0	0	0	0
●★Peanut butter flavor chips, Reese's (¼ cup)	230	19.0	13.0	NA	0	NA
★Pineapple, candied (½ cup)	357	90.4	0.5	0	0	7
Yeast, active dry, Fleischmann's (¼ oz.)	20	3.0	0	0	0	10
Yeast, brewer's (1 Tbsp.)	23	3.1	0.1	0	0	10
Yeast, fresh active, Fleischmann's (0.6 oz.)	15	2.0	0	0	0	5

CONDIMENTS

Food Description	Calories	Carbohydrates (grams)	Fat (grams)	Saturated Fat (grams)	Cholesterol (milligrams)	Sodium (milligrams)
●Bac O's (1 Tbsp.)	40	2.0	2.0	NA	NA	230
●★Catsup, Del Monte (¼ cup)	60	16.0	0	0	0	730
Catsup, imitation, Featherweight (1 Tbsp.)	6	1.0	0	0	0	5
●Catsup mix, imitation, Weight Watchers (2 Tbsp.)	8	2.0	0	0	0	NA
●★Catsup, with salt (1 Tbsp.)	16	3.8	0.1	0	0	156
Chives, chopped (1 Tbsp.)	1	0.2	0	0	0	1
Condiment Sauces						
●★Barbecue, French's (1 Tbsp.)	25	5.0	0	0	0	250
●★Barbecue, hickory smoke flavor, Open Pit (1 Tbsp.)	20	6.0	0	0	0	227
●★Barbecue, Open Pit (1 Tbsp.)	16	4.0	0	0	0	238
●★Barbecue, smoky, French's (1 Tbsp.)	25	5.0	0	0	0	295
●★Chili (1 Tbsp.)	16	3.7	0	0	0	200
Chili, Featherweight (1 Tbsp.)	8	2.0	0	0	0	10
●★Cocktail, Del Monte (¼ cup)	70	17.0	1.0	NA	0	765
●Red pepper sauce, Tabasco (2 oz.)	4	1.0	0	0	0	405
●Soy, La Choy (1 Tbsp.)	8	0.9	0.1	Tr.	Tr.	975
●★Steak, A-1 (1 Tbsp.)	12	3.0	1.0	0	0	275
●★Sweet and sour, Contadina (4 oz.)	120	25.0	2.0	NA	NA	450
●★Sweet and sour, La Choy (½ cup)	262	64.2	0.4	Tr.	Tr.	640
●★Taco, mild, Old El Paso (3½ oz.)	38	8.0	0	0	0	NA

Alerts: ● Sodium ★ Sugar ■ Cholesterol

Food Description	Calories	Carbohydrates (grams)	Fat (grams)	Saturated Fat (grams)	Cholesterol (milligrams)	Sodium (milligrams)
●★Taco, *Ortega* (1 Tbsp.)	22	5.0	1.0	0	0	80
●Tartar, *Hellmann's* (1 Tbsp.)	70	0.2	8.0	1.0	5	180
●Tartar, low calorie (1 Tbsp.)	31	0.9	3.1	0.6	7	99
●Tartar, *Seven Seas* (1 Tbsp.)	80	0	9.0	1.0	NA	125
●Worcestershire, *French's* (1 Tbsp.)	10	2.0	0	0	0	180
●Worcestershire, *Lea & Perrins* (1 tsp.)	4	0.8	Tr.	0	0	40
Garlic, raw (1 clove)	4	0.9	0	0	0	1
Horseradish, prepared (1 Tbsp.)	6	1.4	0	0	0	14
●Mustard, *Brown 'n Spicy, French's* (1 Tbsp.)	15	1.0	1.0	NA	0	150
●Mustard, Dijon, *Grey Poupon* (1 Tbsp.)	18	1.0	1.0	NA	0	445
Mustard, low sodium, *Featherweight* (1 tsp.)	NA	NA	NA	NA	0	1
●Mustard, with horseradish, *French's* (1 Tbsp.)	15	1.0	1.0	NA	0	280
●*Nut O's* (1 Tbsp.)	35	3.0	2.0	NA	NA	55
●Olives, green (10 large)	45	0.5	4.9	0.5	0	927
●Olives, ripe, Ascolano (10 extra large)	61	1.2	6.5	0.7	0	384
●Olives, ripe, Manzanillo (10 extra large)	61	1.2	6.5	0.7	0	384
●Olives, ripe, Mission (10 extra large)	87	1.5	9.5	1.1	0	354
●Olives, ripe, salt cured, Greek style (10 extra large)	89	2.3	9.5	1.0	0	868
●Olives, ripe, Sevillano (10 giant)	64	1.9	6.5	0.7	0	569
●*On Yo's* (1 Tbsp.)	35	3.0	2.0	NA	NA	45
Parsley, chopped (1 Tbsp.)	2	0.3	0	0	0	1
Pickles						
●★Bread and butter, *Fannings* (3.5 oz.)	45	11.5	0.1	0	0	525
●Cucumber, dill (1 medium)	7	1.4	0.1	0	0	928
●Cucumber, fresh (2 slices)	11	2.7	0	0	0	100
Cucumber, sliced, *Featherweight* (1 oz.)	12	3.0	0	0	0	5
●Cucumber, sour (1 medium)	6	1.3	0.1	0	0	879
Dill, *Featherweight* (1 oz.)	4	1.0	0	0	0	5
Dill, kosher, *Featherweight* (1 oz.)	4	1.0	0	0	0	5
●Kosher, *Claussen* (2 oz. pickle)	7	1.2	0.1	0	0	581

Alerts: ● Sodium ★ Sugar ■ Cholesterol

Food Description	Calories	Carbohydrates (grams)	Fat (grams)	Saturated Fat (grams)	Cholesterol (milligrams)	Sodium (milligrams)
●★Sweet and sour, *Claussen* (0.18 oz. slice)	3	0.8	Tr.	0	0	25
●★Sweet, chopped (1 cup)	234	58.4	0.6	0	0	1139
●★Sweet, gherkin (½ oz. pickle)	22	5.5	0.1	0	0	106
Relish, cucumber, unsalted, *Featherweight* (2 Tbsp.)	11	2.3	0	0	0	5
●Relish, pickle (2 tsp.)	14	3.4	0.1	0	0	71
●Sauterne, cooking, *Regina* (¼ cup)	2	1.0	0	0	0	365
Seasonings						
●Chili powder, with seasoning added (1 tsp.)	7	1.1	0.2	0	0	31
●★Coating mix, for chicken, *Shake 'N Bake* (¼ package)	70	10.0	3.0	NA	0	595
●★Coating mix, for fish, *Shake 'N Bake* (¼ package)	60	9.0	2.0	NA	0	535
●★Coating mix, for pork, *Shake 'N Bake* (¼ package)	10	11.0	1.0	NA	0	660
Fish, *Featherweight* (¼ tsp.)	0	0	0	0	0	1
●★Marinade, chicken, dry, *Adolph's* (1 tsp.)	NA	NA	0	0	0	500
Meat, *Featherweight* (¼ tsp.)	0	0	0	0	0	Tr.
●Meat tenderizer, *French's* (1 tsp.)	2	0.5	0.5	0	0	1760
●Meat tenderizer, seasoned, *Adolph's* (1 tsp.)	NA	NA	0	0	0	1880
●Meat tenderizer, steak sauce flavor, *Adolph's* (1 tsp.)	NA	NA	0	0	0	1170
●★Mix, *Chili-O, French's* (1¾ oz.)	25	5.0	0	0	0	630
●★Mix, hamburger, *French's* (1 oz.)	25	5.0	0	0	0	440
●★Mix, sloppy joe, *French's* (1½ oz.)	16	4.0	0	0	0	390
Poultry, *Featherweight* (¼ tsp.)	0	0	0	0	0	Tr.
●Salt (1 tsp.)	0	0	0	0	0	2131
●Salt, celery, *French's* (1 tsp.)	2	0.5	0.5	0	0	1430
●Salt, garlic, *French's* (1 tsp.)	4	1.0	0.5	0	0	1850
●Salt, imitation butter flavor, *French's* (1 tsp.)	8	0	1.0	0	0	1090
●Salt, onion, *French's* (1 tsp.)	1	1.0	0.5	0	0	1620
Salt substitute, garlic, *Featherweight* (¼ tsp.)	0	0	0	0	0	Tr.
Salt substitute, seasoned, dietetic, *McCormick* (1 tsp.)	0	0	0	0	0	1

Alerts: ● Sodium ★ Sugar ■ Cholesterol

Food Description	Calories	Carbohydrates (grams)	Fat (grams)	Saturated Fat (grams)	Cholesterol (milligrams)	Sodium (milligrams)
Salt substitute, seasoned, *Featherweight* (¼ tsp.)	0	0	0	0	0	Tr.
• Sherry, cooking, *Regina* (¼ cup)	20	5.0	0	0	0	370
Vinegar, cider (1 Tbsp.)	2	0.9	0	0	0	0
Vinegar, distilled (1 Tbsp.)	2.0	0.8	0	0	0	0
Vinegar, red wine, *Regina* (1 oz.)	4	1.0	0	0	0	5

Cookies

•★Almond windmill, *Nabisco* (3 cookies)	140	21.0	5.0	NA	NA	NA
•★Apple crisp, *Nabisco* (3 cookies)	150	21.0	6.0	NA	NA	NA
•★Brownie, *Hostess* (1¼ oz.)	150	24.0	6.0	NA	11	75
•★Brownie, with icing, frozen (0.9 oz.)	103	14.9	5.0	1.7	10	49
•★■Brownie, with icing, frozen, *Sara Lee* (⅛ package)	192	26.0	9.7	NA	NA	108
•★Brownie, with nuts, homemade (1¾" square)	97	10.2	6.3	1.4	17	50
•★Brown sugar, *Pepperidge Farm* (3 cookies)	150	21.0	7.0	NA	NA	73
•★Butter flavor, *Nabisco* (6 cookies)	140	21.0	5.0	NA	NA	NA
•★Butter, packaged (10 cookies)	229	35.4	8.4	4.0	38	209
•★Cameo creme sandwich, *Nabisco* (2 cookies)	140	21.0	5.0	NA	NA	NA
•★Capri, *Pepperidge Farm* (2 cookies)	170	20.0	10.0	NA	NA	77
•★Caramel peanut log, *Heyday* (1 cookie)	120	13.0	7.0	NA	NA	NA
•★Chocolate cakes, *Mallomar* (2 cookies)	120	17.0	5.0	NA	NA	NA
•★Chocolate chip, *Chips Ahoy* (3 cookies)	160	21.0	7.0	NA	NA	NA
•★■Chocolate chip, homemade (4 cookies)	206	24.0	12.0	3.4	20	139

Alerts: • Sodium ★ Sugar ■ Cholesterol

Food Description	Calories	Carbohydrates (grams)	Fat (grams)	Saturated Fat (grams)	Cholesterol (milligrams)	Sodium (milligrams)
●★Chocolate chip, packaged (10 medium cookies)	344	50.9	15.3	4.7	28	292
★Chocolate chip, *Pepperidge Farm* (3 cookies)	130	17.0	6.0	NA	NA	40
Chocolate creme wafers, *Featherweight* (1 wafer)	40	4.0	2.0	NA	NA	14
Chocolate crescent, *Featherweight* (1 cookie)	40	4.0	2.0	NA	NA	6
●★Chocolate sandwich, *Oreo* (3 cookies)	150	22.0	7.0	NA	NA	NA
●★Chocolate wafers, *Famous, Nabisco* (5 wafers)	140	23.0	4.0	NA	NA	NA
●★Cinnamon sugar, *Pepperidge Farm* (3 cookies)	160	21.0	7.0	NA	NA	93
●★■Coconut bars (10 cookies)	445	57.5	22.0	8.4	98	133
●★Coconut bars, *Bakers Bonus, Nabisco* (3 cookies)	130	16.0	6.0	NA	NA	NA
●★Coconut chocolate chip, *Nabisco* (2 cookies)	150	18.0	8.0	NA	NA	NA
●★Coconut granola, *Kitchen Hearth, Pepperidge Farm* (3 cookies)	170	31.0	9.0	NA	NA	98
●★Creme sandwich, *Mayfair English Style Assortment, Nabisco* (2 cookies)	130	18.0	6.0	NA	NA	NA
●★Creme wafer sticks, *Nabisco* (3 wafers)	140	19.0	7.0	NA	NA	NA
●★Fig bars, *Fig Newton* (2 bars)	120	22.0	2.0	NA	NA	NA
●★Fig bars, packaged (4 bars)	200	42.2	3.1	0.9	22	141
●★Fudge and butterscotch chip, *Bakers Bonus, Nabisco* (2 cookies)	160	22.0	7.0	NA	NA	NA
●★Fudge chip, *Pepperidge Farm* (3 cookies)	170	22.0	8.0	NA	NA	105
●★Fudge/fudge-creme sandwich, *Nabisco* (3 cookies)	160	23.0	7.0	NA	NA	NA
●★Ginger snaps, Old Fashion, *Nabisco* (4 cookies)	120	22.0	3.0	NA	NA	NA
●★Ginger snaps, packaged (10 cookies)	294	55.9	6.2	1.6	27	399
Lemon flavor, *Featherweight* (1 cookie)	40	4.0	2.0	NA	NA	3
●★Lemon nut crunch, *Pepperidge Farm* (3 cookies)	180	20.0	10.0	NA	NA	68
●★Lido, *Pepperidge Farm* (2 cookies)	190	20.0	11.0	NA	NA	64

Alerts: ● Sodium ★ Sugar ■ Cholesterol

Food Description	Calories	Carbohydrates (grams)	Fat (grams)	Saturated Fat (grams)	Cholesterol (milligrams)	Sodium (milligrams)
★■ Macaroons, packaged (2 cookies)	181	25.1	8.8	6.1	41	12
●★■ Marshmallow, chocolate coated, packaged (4 cookies)	213	37.6	6.9	4.2	40	108
●★■ Marshmallow, coconut coated, packaged (4 cookies)	294	52.1	9.5	5.8	55	150
●★ Marshmallow sandwich, *Nabisco* (4 cookies)	120	23.0	3.0	NA	NA	NA
●★ Milano, *Pepperidge Farm* (3 cookies)	190	22.0	11.0	NA	NA	63
●★■ Molasses (3 cookies)	137	24.7	3.4	0.9	13	125
●★ Molasses crisps, *Pepperidge Farm* (3 cookies)	90	13.0	4.0	NA	NA	56
●★ Molasses, *Nabisco Pantry* (2 cookies)	120	19.0	4.0	NA	NA	NA
●★ Nassau, *Pepperdige Farm* (2 cookies)	150	16.0	9.0	NA	NA	60
●★ Oatmeal, *Bakers Bonus, Nabisco* (2 cookies)	160	24.0	6.0	NA	NA	NA
●★ Oatmeal raisin, *Pepperidge Farm* (3 cookies)	170	23.0	8.0	NA	NA	159
●★ Oatmeal, with raisins, packaged (4 large cookies)	235	38.2	8.0	2.1	20	84
★ Orleans, *Pepperidge Farm* (3 cookies)	100	11.0	6.0	NA	NA	22
Peanut butter creme wafers, *Featherweight* (1 wafer)	40	4.0	2.0	NA	NA	14
●★ Peanut butter sandwich, *Nutter Butter* (2 cookies)	140	18.0	6.0	NA	NA	NA
●★ Peanut creme patties, *Nabisco* (4 cookies)	140	15.0	7.0	NA	NA	NA
★ Peanut, *Pepperidge Farm* (3 cookies)	140	16.0	7.0	NA	NA	56
●★ Peanut sandwich, packaged (4 cookies)	232	32.8	9.4	2.0	19	84
★ Pirouette, *Pepperidge Farm* (3 cookies)	120	14.0	7.0	NA	NA	38
●★ Sandwich, chocolate or vanilla, packaged (4 cookies)	198	27.7	9.0	2.4	16	193
Sandwich creme, *Featherweight* (1 cookie)	50	6.0	2.0	NA	NA	3
●★ Sandwich, *Mystic Mint* (2 cookies)	180	22.0	9.0	NA	NA	NA
●★ Shortbread, *Lorna Doone* (4 cookies)	160	20.0	8.0	NA	NA	NA

Alerts: ● Sodium ★ Sugar ■ Cholesterol

Food Description	Calories	Carbohydrates (grams)	Fat (grams)	Saturated Fat (grams)	Cholesterol (milligrams)	Sodium (milligrams)
★Shortbread, packaged (10 cookies)	374	48.8	17.3	4.3	29	45
●★Shortbread, *Pepperidge Farm* (2 cookies)	130	15.0	8.0	NA	NA	69
●★Shortcake, *Melt-A-Way* (2 cookies)	140	16.0	7.0	NA	NA	NA
●★Sugar, homemade (10 cookies)	355	54.4	13.4	3.6	31	254
●★Sugar, *Pepperidge Farm* (3 cookies)	160	21.0	7.0	NA	NA	91
●★Sugar wafers, *Biscos* (3 wafers)	150	20.0	7.0	NA	NA	NA
●★Sugar wafers, packaged (10 large wafers)	461	69.7	18.4	4.7	37	179
●★Sunflower raisin, *Pepperidge Farm* (3 cookies)	160	18.0	9.0	NA	NA	236
Vanilla creme wafers, *Featherweight* (1 wafer)	40	4.0	2.0	NA	NA	14
Vanilla, *Featherweight* (1 wafer)	40	4.0	2.0	NA	NA	14
●★Vanilla wafers, *Nilla, Nabisco* (7 wafers)	130	21.0	4.0	NA	NA	NA
★Vanilla wafers, packaged (10 small wafers)	139	22.3	4.8	1.2	12	75
COOKIE DOUGHS						
●★Brownie, fudge, *Pillsbury Slice N Bake* (1 brownie)	130	21.0	5.0	NA	NA	140
●★Chocolate chip, *Mrs. Goodcookie* (3 cookies)	170	23.0	7.0	3.0	10	60
●★Chocolate chip, *Pillsbury Slice N Bake* (3 cookies)	160	22.0	8.0	NA	NA	125
●★Chocolate fudge, *Mrs. Goodcookie* (3 cookies)	170	22.0	8.0	2.0	10	80
●★Oatmeal, *Pillsbury Slice N Bake* (3 cookies)	170	22.0	8.0	NA	NA	130
●★Oatmeal raisin, *Mrs. Goodcookie* (3 cookies)	160	22.0	7.0	2.0	10	140
●★Peanut butter, *Mrs. Goodcookie* (3 cookies)	180	19.0	10.0	2.0	10	100
●★Peanut butter, *Pillsbury Slice N Bake* (3 cookies)	160	19.0	9.0	NA	NA	235
●★Plain, chilled (4 cookies)	238	31.2	12.0	3.0	19	263
●★Sugar, *Mrs. Goodcookie* (3 cookies)	160	22.0	7.0	2.0	10	90
●★Sugar, *Pillsbury Slice N Bake* (3 cookies)	190	25.0	9.0	NA	NA	230

Alerts: ● Sodium ★ Sugar ■ Cholesterol

Food Description	Calories	Carbohydrates (grams)	Fat (grams)	Saturated Fat (grams)	Cholesterol (milligrams)	Sodium (milligrams)
COOKIE MIXES						
Brownie						
●★Chocolate chip/butterscotch, *Betty Crocker* (1/16 package)	130	21.0	5.0	NA	NA	120
●★Double fudge, *Duncan Hines* (1/24 family-size package)	130	19.0	5.0	1.3	NA	100
●★Fudge, *Betty Crocker* (1/24 family-size package)	110	21.0	2.0	NA	NA	90
●★Fudge, *Betty Crocker Supreme* (1/24 package)	120	21.0	3.0	NA	NA	70
●★Fudge, *Jiffy* (1/12 package)	80	13.7	2.4	NA	NA	NA
●★Fudge, *Pillsbury Deluxe* (1/24 family-size package)	110	21.0	2.0	NA	NA	100
●★German chocolate, *Betty Crocker* (1/16 package)	150	26.0	5.0	NA	NA	80
●★*Nestle* (1 oz.)	130	21.0	4.0	NA	NA	80
●★Walnut, *Pillsbury* (1/24 family-size package)	120	21.0	4.0	NA	NA	100
●★With nuts, prepared (1¾" square brownie)	86	12.6	4.0	0.9	9	33
★Butter, dietetic, *Batter-Lite* (mix for 2 cookies)	40	7.0	1.0	NA	NA	6
●★Chocolate chip, *Big Batch* (mix for 2 cookies)	150	18.0	8.0	NA	NA	75
●★Chocolate chip, *Quaker Oats* (mix for 2 cookies)	100	17.0	3.0	NA	NA	NA
●★Chocolate, dietetic, *Batter-Lite* (mix for 2 cookies)	45	7.0	1.0	NA	Tr.	40
★Coconut macaroon, *Betty Crocker* (1/24 package)	80	10.0	4.0	NA	NA	15
●★Date bar, *Betty Crocker* (1/32 package)	60	9.0	2.0	NA	NA	35
●★Double chocolate, *Betty Crocker Big Batch* (mix for 2 cookies)	120	17.0	6.0	NA	NA	65
●★Double chocolate, *Duncan Hines* (mix for 2 cookies)	130	18.0	1.0	Tr.	0	75
●★Golden sugar, *Duncan Hines* (mix for 2 cookies)	130	17.0	6.0	NA	0	65
●★Oatmeal, *Quaker Oats* (mix for 2 cookies)	130	19.0	6.0	NA	NA	NA
●★Oatmeal raisin, *Duncan Hines* (mix for 2 cookies)	130	18.0	6.0	1.4	0	70
●★Peanut butter flavored chip, *Betty Crocker Big Batch* (mix for 2 cookies)	120	16.0	6.0	NA	NA	70

Alerts: ● Sodium ★ Sugar ■ Cholesterol

Food Description	Calories	Carbohydrates (grams)	Fat (grams)	Saturated Fat (grams)	Cholesterol (milligrams)	Sodium (milligrams)
●★Plain, prepared (10 cookies)	276	36.4	13.6	3.4	32	194
●★Sugar, *Betty Crocker Big Batch* (mix for 2 cookies)	120	18.0	5.0	NA	NA	70
●★Vienna Dream bar, *Betty Crocker* (1/24 package)	80	10.0	4.0	NA	NA	50

Crackers

Food Description	Calories	Carbohydrates (grams)	Fat (grams)	Saturated Fat (grams)	Cholesterol (milligrams)	Sodium (milligrams)
●★Animal (10 crackers)	112	20.8	2.4	0.6	0	78
●★Animal, *Barnum's, Nabisco* (11 crackers)	130	21.0	4.0	NA	0	NA
●★*Bacon 'N Dip* (17 crackers)	150	16.0	8.0	NA	NA	NA
●★Butter, circles (10 crackers)	151	22.2	5.9	2.0	0	360
●★Cheddar, sticks, *Pepperidge Farm* (1 oz.)	120	19.0	5.0	NA	NA	370
●Cheddar triangles, *Nabisco* (17 crackers)	150	16.0	8.0	NA	NA	NA
●Cheese (1.1 oz.)	150	18.9	6.7	2.6	10	325
●★*Chicken in a Biskit* (14 crackers)	150	16.0	9.0	NA	NA	NA
●*Dip in a Chip* (15 crackers)	150	16.0	8.0	NA	NA	NA
●★*Escort* (7 crackers)	150	18.0	8.0	NA	NA	NA
●★French onion, *Nabisco* (12 crackers)	150	18.0	7.0	NA	NA	NA
●*Goldfish*, cheddar cheese (1/4 oz.)	35	4.0	2.0	NA	NA	75
●*Goldfish*, lightly salted (1/4 oz.)	35	4.0	2.0	NA	NA	55
●*Goldfish*, parmesan (1/4 oz.)	35	4.0	2.0	NA	NA	95
●*Goldfish*, pizza (1/4 oz.)	35	4.0	2.0	NA	NA	80
●*Goldfish*, pretzel (1/4 oz.)	30	5.0	1.0	NA	NA	125
Graham Crackers						
●★Chocolate-coated (0.5 oz. cracker)	62	8.8	3.1	0.9	0	52
●★Chocolate-coated, *Nabisco* (3 crackers)	170	21.0	8.0	NA	0	NA
●★Crumbs (1 cup)	326	62.3	8.0	1.9	0	569
●★Crumbs, *Nabisco* (0.6 oz.)	70	12.0	2.0	NA	0	NA
●★*Honey Maid* (4 crackers)	120	22.0	3.0	NA	0	NA

Alerts: ● Sodium ★ Sugar ■ Cholesterol

Food Description	Calories	Carbohydrates (grams)	Fat (grams)	Saturated Fat (grams)	Cholesterol (milligrams)	Sodium (milligrams)
●★Honey, *Schulze and Burch* (2 crackers)	115	20.0	3.0	NA	0	NA
●★Party, *Nabisco* (3 crackers)	140	18.0	7.0	NA	0	NA
●★Plain (0.5 oz. cracker)	55	10.4	1.3	0.3	0	95
●★Sugar honey (0.5 oz. cracker)	58	10.8	1.6	0.4	0	71
●★Sugar honey, crumbs (1 cup)	349	64.9	9.7	2.3	0	428
●★Sugar honey, *Fireside, Nabisco* (4 crackers)	120	21.0	3.0	NA	0	NA
Matzos, *Manischewitz* (1 cracker)	90	20.0	0	0	0	10
Matzo, miniature, *Manischewitz* (1 cracker)	9	2.0	0	0	0	10
Matzos, no salt, *Streit's* (1 cracker)	100	23.0	0.5	Tr.	0	2
Matzos, unsalted, *Goodman* (1 cracker)	130	26.0	1.0	NA	0	10
Matzos, wheat, *Manischewitz* (1 cracker)	8	2.0	0	0	0	10
●★Pumpernickel, sticks, *Pepperidge Farm* (1 oz.)	110	17.0	4.0	NA	NA	351
●★*Ritz* (9 crackers)	150	18.0	8.0	NA	NA	NA
●*Roman Meal Wafers* (1 oz. or 8 crackers)	120	20.0	3.0	NA	Tr.	NA
●Rye, whole-grain (10 crackers)	224	49.6	0.8	0	1	573
●*Sea Rounds* (2 crackers)	90	15.0	2.0	NA	NA	NA
●Sesame, butter flavored, *Nabisco* (9 crackers)	150	17.0	8.0	NA	NA	NA
●★Sesame, sticks, *Pepperidge Farm* (1 oz.)	120	16.0	5.0	NA	NA	337
●★*Sesame Wheats* (9 crackers)	150	16.0	9.0	NA	NA	NA
●★*Sociables* (14 crackers)	150	18.0	7.0	NA	NA	NA
Soda Crackers						
●Crumbs (1 cup)	307	49.4	9.2	2.2	0	770
●★*Oysterette* (36 crackers)	120	20.0	3.0	NA	0	NA
●Regular (10 crackers)	221	35.6	6.6	1.6	0	554
●Saltine (10 crackers)	123	20.3	3.4	0.8	0	312
●Saltine, crumbs (1 cup)	303	50.1	8.4	2.0	0	770
●Saltine, *Premium, Nabisco* (10 crackers)	120	20.0	4.0	NA	0	NA
Unsalted, *Featherweight* (4 crackers)	10	10.0	2.0	NA	0	10
●Unsalted tops, *Premium, Nabisco* (10 crackers)	120	20.0	4.0	NA	0	NA
●Swiss cheese flavored, *Nabisco* (15 crackers)	150	17.0	8.0	NA	NA	NA

Alerts: ● Sodium ★ Sugar ■ Cholesterol

Food Description	Calories	Carbohydrates (grams)	Fat (grams)	Saturated Fat (grams)	Cholesterol (milligrams)	Sodium (milligrams)
●*Tid-Bit* (32 crackers)	150	16.0	9.0	NA	NA	NA
●*Triscuit* (7 crackers)	140	21.0	5.0	NA	NA	NA
●★*Vegetable Thins* (13 crackers)	150	17.0	8.0	NA	NA	NA
●★*Waverly Wafers* (8 crackers)	140	21.0	6.0	NA	NA	NA
●★*Wheatsworth* (9 crackers)	130	16.0	6.0	NA	0	NA
●★*Wheat Thins, Nabisco* (16 crackers)	140	19.0	6.0	NA	NA	NA
●★Whole wheat, sticks, *Pepperidge Farm* (1 oz.)	110	17.0	4.0	NA	NA	366
TOASTS						
● Bran, *Ideal Flat Bread* (1 slice)	19	4.1	Tr.	0	0	47
● Brown, *King's Bread* (2 slices)	90	20.0	0	0	0	NA
● Dark, *Finn Crisp* (4 slices)	80	17.0	0	0	0	NA
● Light, *Finn Crisp* (4 slices)	80	15.0	Tr.	Tr.	0	NA
● Light, *King's Bread* (2 slices)	70	15.0	0	0	0	NA
Melba Toast						
● Garlic flavor, *Old London* (5 rounds)	50	9.0	1.0	NA	0	NA
● Onion flavor, *Old London* (5 rounds)	50	9.0	1.0	NA	0	NA
● Rye, *Devonsheer* (1 slice)	16	3.0	0	0	0	NA
● Rye flavor, *Old London* (5 rounds)	50	9.0	1.0	NA	0	NA
● Rye, *Wasa Lite* (1 slice)	30	6.0	0.2	0	0	20
● Sesame, *Devonsheer* (1 slice)	16	3.0	0	NA	0	NA
● Sesame flavor, *Old London* (5 rounds)	10	8.0	2.0	NA	0	NA
● Wheat, *Devonsheer* (1 slice)	16	3.0	0	0	0	NA
● Rye, golden, *Wasa Crisp* (1 slice)	37	8.0	0.2	0	0	43
● Rye, hearty, *Wasa Crisp* (1 slice)	54	11.0	0.3	0	0	38
● Rye, mora, *Wasa Crisp* (3.2 oz. slice)	333	70.5	1.5	0	0	514
● Rye, *RyKrisp* (2 triple crackers)	50	10.0	0	0	0	110
● Rye, *RyKrisp,* seasoned (2 triple crackers)	60	9.0	1.0	0	0	220
●★Rusk (1 cracker)	38	6.4	0.8	0.2	1	22
●★Rusk, Holland, *Nabisco* (2 crackers)	80	15.0	2.0	NA	NA	NA
●★Sesame, *Meal Mates* (6 crackers)	130	19.0	5.0	NA	NA	NA
● Sesame, *Wasa Crisp* (1 slice)	54	11.0	0.3	0	0	38
● Sport, *Wasa Crisp* (1 slice)	43	9.0	1.0	0	0	66

Alerts: ● Sodium ★ Sugar ■ Cholesterol

Food Description	Calories	Carbohydrates (grams)	Fat (grams)	Saturated Fat (grams)	Cholesterol (milligrams)	Sodium (milligrams)
• Ultra thin, *Ideal Flat Bread* (1 slice)	12	3.0	0.1	0	0	25
• Whole grain, *Ideal Flat Bread* (1 slice)	19	4.0	0.1	0	0	47
• Zwieback (1 piece)	30	5.2	0.6	0.2	1	18

Cream and Yogurt

CREAM AND CREAM SUBSTITUTES						
■ Cream, half and half, 11.7% fat (1 Tbsp.)	20	0.7	1.8	1.0	6	6
■ Cream, half and half, *Land O' Lakes* (1 Tbsp.)	20	1.0	2.0	1.0	6	6
■ Cream, heavy, 37.6% fat (1 Tbsp.)	53	0.5	5.6	3.1	20	5
■ Cream, light, 20.6% fat (1 Tbsp.)	32	0.6	3.1	1.7	10	6
■ Cream, sour (1 Tbsp.)	26	0.5	2.5	1.6	5	6
■ Cream, sour, half and half (1 Tbsp.)	20	0.6	1.8	1.1	6	6
Cream, sour, imitation, nondairy (2 Tbsp.)	59	1.9	5.5	5.0	0	29
• Cream, sour, imitation, *Pet* (1 Tbsp.)	25	1.0	2.0	NA	1	NA
• Cream substitute, *Milnot* (½ cup)	150	12.0	8.0	NA	5	NA
Cream substitute, nondairy, *Coffee Rich* (½ oz.)	20	2.1	1.4	0.9	0	7
Cream substitute, nondairy, dry, *Coffee-Mate* (1 tsp.)	16	1.7	1.0	NA	Tr.	5
Cream substitute, nondairy, dry, *Pet* (1 tsp.)	10	1.0	1.0	NA	NA	NA
Cream, whipped, pressurized (1 Tbsp.)	8	0.4	0.7	0.4	2	4
■ Cream, whipping, *Land O' Lakes* (1 Tbsp.)	45	0	5.0	3.0	17	5
■ Cream, whipping, light, 31.3% fat (1 Tbsp.)	45	0.5	4.7	2.6	17	5

Alerts: • Sodium ★ Sugar ■ Cholesterol

Food Description	Calories	Carbohydrates (grams)	Fat (grams)	Saturated Fat (grams)	Cholesterol (milligrams)	Sodium (milligrams)
• Whey (1 cup)	64	12.5	0.7	0	5	196
YOGURT						
•★ Low fat, all fruit flavors (except lemon), *Dannon* (1 cup)	260	49.0	3.0	NA	20	250
•★ Low fat, coffee, vanilla and lemon, *Dannon* (1 cup)	200	32.0	4.0	NA	15	255
•★ Low fat, frozen, all fruit flavors (except lemon), *Danny In-A-Cup, Dannon* (8 oz.)	210	42.0	2.0	NA	10	70
★ Low fat, frozen, chocolate coated, all flavors, *Danny On-A-Stick, Dannon* (1 bar)	140	15.0	8.0	NA	5	15
★ Low fat, frozen, *Danny Parfait, Dannon* (4 oz.)	160	35.0	1.0	NA	5	15
•★ Low fat, frozen, lemon, *Danny In-A-Cup, Dannon* (8 oz.)	180	20.0	2.0	NA	10	70
•★ Low fat, frozen on a stick, chocolate coated, *Tuscan Pops* (1 bar)	150	17.0	8.0	NA	NA	NA
•★ Low fat, frozen on a stick, chocolate, *Tuscan Pops* (1 bar)	85	16.0	1.0	NA	NA	NA
★ Low fat, frozen, uncoated, all flavors, *Danny On-A-Stick, Dannon* (1 bar)	70	15.0	1.0	NA	5	15
• Low fat, plain, *Dannon* (1 cup)	150	17.0	4.0	NA	15	235
• Low fat, plain (from partially skimmed milk) (8 oz.)	144	16.0	3.5	2.3	14	159
•★ Nonfat, all fruit flavors, *Sweet 'N Low* (8 oz.)	150	32.0	0	0	NA	170
• Nonfat, plain, *Sweet 'N Low* (8 oz.)	90	15.0	0	0	NA	160
•★ Regular, all fruit flavors, *Yoplait* (6 oz.)	200	32.0	5.0	NA	NA	NA
• Regular, plain (from whole milk) (1 cup)	152	12.0	8.3	4.6	20	15
• Regular, plain, *Yoplait* (6 oz.)	130	12.0	5.0	NA	NA	NA

Alerts: • Sodium ★ Sugar ■ Cholesterol

Fast Foods

Food Description	Calories	Carbohydrates (grams)	Fat (grams)	Saturated Fat (grams)	Cholesterol (milligrams)	Sodium (milligrams)
●★ Banana split, *Dairy Queen* (1 serving)	540	91.0	15.0	NA	30	NA
●★■ *Big Mac, McDonald's* (average serving)	563	40.6	33.0	NA	86	1010
●★■ Cheeseburger, *Burger King* (1 sandwich)	350	30.0	17.0	NA	NA	730
●★■ Cheeseburger, double, *Burger King* (1 sandwich)	530	32.0	31.0	NA	NA	990
●★■ Cheeseburger, double, *Wendy's* (1 serving)	800	41.0	48.0	NA	155	1414
●★■ Cheeseburger, *McDonald's* (average serving)	307	29.8	14.1	NA	37	767
●★■ Cheeseburger, triple, *Wendy's* (1 serving)	1040	35.0	68.0	NA	225	1848
●★■ Cheeseburger, *Wendy's* (1 serving)	580	34.0	34.0	NA	90	1085
●■ Chicken, side breast, *Crispy Recipe, Kentucky Fried Chicken* (1 piece)	286	14.4	17.8	NA	55	477
●■ Chicken, side breast, *Original Recipe, Kentucky Fried Chicken* (1 piece)	198	7.1	11.7	NA	48	385
●■ Chicken, thigh, *Crispy Recipe, Kentucky Fried Chicken* (1 piece)	343	12.6	23.3	NA	117	587
●■ Chicken, thigh, *Original Recipe, Kentucky Fried Chicken* (1 piece)	257	6.5	17.5	NA	96	498
●★■ Chicken, 2-piece dinner with potato and gravy, slaw, and roll, *Crispy Recipe, Kentucky Fried Chicken*	902	58.4	50.0	NA	176	1529
●★■ Chicken, 2-piece dinner with potato and gravy, slaw, and roll, *Original Recipe, Kentucky Fried Chicken*	661	47.8	37.8	NA	172	1536

Alerts: ● Sodium ★ Sugar ■ Cholesterol

Food Description	Calories	Carbohydrates (grams)	Fat (grams)	Saturated Fat (grams)	Cholesterol (milligrams)	Sodium (milligrams)
●★■ Chili, *Wendy's* (1 serving)	230	21.0	8.0	NA	25	1065
●★ Cole slaw, *Kentucky Fried Chicken* (1 serving)	122	7.5	12.7	NA	7	205
●★■ Cookies, chocolate chip, *McDonald's* (1 serving)	342	44.8	16.3	NA	18	313
●★ Cookies, *McDonaldland* (1 serving)	308	48.7	10.8	NA	10	358
●★ Dilly Bar, *Dairy Queen* (1 bar)	240	22.0	15.0	NA	10	NA
★ Dinner roll, *Kentucky Fried Chicken* (1 roll)	61	10.9	1.1	NA	Tr.	24
●★ DQ Sandwich, *Dairy Queen* (1 sandwich)	140	24.0	4.0	NA	10	NA
●■ Egg McMuffin, *McDonald's* (average serving)	327	31.0	14.8	NA	229	885
● English Muffin with butter, *McDonald's* (average serving)	186	29.5	5.3	NA	13	318
●■ Filet-O-Fish, *McDonald's* (average serving)	432	37.4	25.0	NA	47	781
●★ Float, *Dairy Queen* (1 float)	330	59.0	8.0	NA	20	NA
●★ Float, *Mr. Misty, Dairy Queen* (1 float)	440	85.0	8.0	NA	20	NA
●★ Freeze, *Dairy Queen* (1 freeze)	520	89.0	13.0	NA	35	NA
●★ Freeze, *Mr. Misty, Dairy Queen* (1 freeze)	500	87.0	12.0	NA	35	NA
●■ French fries, regular, *Burger King* (2.4 oz. serving)	210	25.0	11.0	NA	NA	230
●■ French fries, regular, *McDonald's* (average serving)	220	26.1	11.5	NA	9	109
● French fries, *Wendy's* (1 serving)	330	41.0	16.0	NA	5	112
● Gravy, *Kentucky Fried Chicken* (1 serving)	23	1.3	1.8	NA	Tr.	81
●★ Hamburger, *Burger King* (1 sandwich)	290	29.0	13.0	NA	NA	525
●★■ Hamburger, *Double Beef Whopper, Burger King* (1 hamburger)	850	52.0	52.0	NA	NA	1080
●★■ Hamburger, *Double Beef Whopper with Cheese, Burger King* (1 hamburger)	950	54.0	60.0	NA	NA	1535
●★■ Hamburger, double, *Wendy's* (1 serving)	670	34.0	40.0	NA	125	980

Alerts: ● Sodium ★ Sugar ■ Cholesterol

Food Description	Calories	Carbohydrates (grams)	Fat (grams)	Saturated Fat (grams)	Cholesterol (milligrams)	Sodium (milligrams)
●★ Hamburger, *McDonald's* (average serving)	255	29.5	9.8	NA	25	520
●★■ Hamburger, single, *Wendy's* (1 serving)	470	34.0	26.0	NA	70	774
●★■ Hamburger, triple, *Wendy's* (1 serving)	850	33.0	51.0	NA	205	1217
●★■ Hamburger, *Whopper, Burger King* (1 hamburger)	630	50.0	36.0	NA	NA	990
●★■ Hamburger, *Whopper Junior, Burger King* (1 hamburger)	370	31.0	20.0	NA	NA	560
●★■ Hamburger, *Whopper Junior with Cheese, Burger King* (1 hamburger)	420	32.0	25.0	NA	NA	785
●★■ Hamburger, *Whopper with Cheese, Burger King* (1 hamburger)	740	52.0	45.0	NA	NA	1405
● Hash brown potatoes, *McDonald's* (average serving)	125	14.0	7.0	NA	7	325
●★■ Hotcakes with butter and syrup, *McDonald's* (average serving)	500	93.9	10.3	NA	47	1070
●★ Ice cream cone, chocolate dipped, large, *Dairy Queen* (1 cone)	450	58.0	20.0	NA	30	NA
●★ Ice cream cone, chocolate dipped, regular, *Dairy Queen* (1 cone)	300	40.0	13.0	NA	20	NA
●★ Ice cream cone, chocolate dipped, small, *Dairy Queen* (1 cone)	150	20.0	7.0	NA	10	NA
●★ Ice cream cone, large, *Dairy Queen* (1 cone)	340	52.0	10.0	NA	30	NA
●★ Ice cream cone, regular, *Dairy Queen* (1 cone)	230	35.0	7.0	NA	20	NA
●★ Ice cream cone, small, *Dairy Queen* (1 cone)	110	18.0	3.0	NA	10	NA
●★■ Ice cream, soft serve, *Frosty, Wendy's* (1 serving)	390	54.0	16.0	NA	45	247
●★■ Malt, chocolate, large, *Dairy Queen* (1 malt)	840	125.0	28.0	NA	70	NA
●★■ Malt, chocolate, regular, *Dairy Queen* (1 malt)	600	89.0	20.0	NA	50	NA
●★■ Malt, chocolate, small, *Dairy Queen* (1 malt)	340	51.0	11.0	NA	30	NA

Alerts: ● Sodium ★ Sugar ■ Cholesterol

Food Description	Calories	Carbohydrates (grams)	Fat (grams)	Saturated Fat (grams)	Cholesterol (milligrams)	Sodium (milligrams)
★Mr. Misty Kiss, Dairy Queen (1 kiss)	70	17.0	0	NA	0	NA
●■ Onion rings, regular, Burger King (2.7 oz. serving)	270	29.0	16.0	NA	NA	450
●★ Parfait, Dairy Queen (1 parfait)	460	81.0	11.0	NA	30	NA
●★■ Pie, apple, Burger King (3 oz. pie)	240	32.0	12.0	NA	NA	335
●★■ Pie, apple, McDonald's (1 pie)	253	29.3	14.3	NA	12	398
●★■ Pie, cherry, McDonald's (1 pie)	260	32.1	13.6	NA	13	427
● Potatoes, Kentucky Fried Chicken (1 serving)	65	12.2	0.9	NA	Tr.	228
●★■ Quarter Pounder, McDonald's (average serving)	424	32.7	21.7	NA	67	735
●★■ Quarter Pounder with Cheese, McDonald's (average serving)	524	32.2	30.7	NA	96	1236
●■ Sausage, McDonald's (average serving)	206	0.6	18.6	NA	43	615
●■ Scrambled eggs, McDonald's (average serving)	180	2.5	13.0	NA	349	205
●★■ Shake, chocolate, Burger King (1 shake)	340	57.0	10.0	NA	NA	280
●★■ Shake, chocolate, McDonald's (1 shake)	383	65.5	9.0	NA	30	300
●★■ Shake, vanilla, Burger King (1 shake)	340	52.0	11.0	NA	NA	320
●★■ Shake, vanilla, McDonald's (1 shake)	352	59.6	8.4	NA	31	201
●★■ Sundae, caramel, McDonald's (1 sundae)	329	52.5	10.0	NA	26	196
●★ Sundae, chocolate, large, Dairy Queen (1 sundae)	400	71.0	9.0	NA	30	NA
●★ Sundae, chocolate, regular, Dairy Queen (1 sundae)	290	51.0	7.0	NA	20	NA
●★ Sundae, chocolate, small, Dairy Queen (1 sundae)	170	30.0	4.0	NA	15	NA
●★ Sundae, Fiesta, Dairy Queen (1 sundae)	570	84.0	22.0	NA	25	NA
●★■ Sundae, hot fudge, McDonald's (1 sundae)	310	46.2	10.0	NA	18	175
●★■ Sundae, strawberry, McDonald's (1 sundae)	289	46.1	8.7	NA	20	96

Alerts: ● Sodium ★ Sugar ■ Cholesterol

Fats, Oils, and Shortenings

Food Description	Calories	Carbohydrates (grams)	Fat (grams)	Saturated Fat (grams)	Cholesterol (milligrams)	Sodium (milligrams)
■ Lard (1 Tbsp.)	117	0	13.0	4.9	12	0
Oils						
Corn, *Mazola* (1 Tbsp.)	120	0	14.0	2.0	0	0
Cottonseed (1 Tbsp.)	120	0	13.6	3.4	0	0
Olive (1 Tbsp.)	119	0	13.5	1.5	0	0
Peanut, *Planters* (1 Tbsp.)	130	0	14.0	2.0	0	0
Popcorn, *Planters* (1 Tbsp.)	130	0	14.0	2.0	0	0
Safflower, *Hollywood* (1 Tbsp.)	120	0	14.0	1.0	0	0
Sesame (1 Tbsp.)	120	0	13.6	1.9	0	0
Soybean (1 Tbsp.)	120	0	13.6	2.0	0	0
Sunflower, *Sunlite* (1 Tbsp.)	120	0	14.0	2.0	0	0
Vegetable, *Crisco* (1 Tbsp.)	120	0	14.0	2.0	0	0
Vegetable, *Puritan* (1 Tbsp.)	120	0	14.0	2.0	0	0
Wesson (1 Tbsp.)	120	0	14.0	3.0	0	0
Shortening, *Snowdrift* (1 Tbsp.)	110	0	12.0	4.0	0	0
Shortening, *Spry* (1 Tbsp.)	93	0	10.5	2.9	0	0
Shortening, vegetable, *Crisco* (1 Tbsp.)	110	0	12.0	3.0	0	0
Vegetable cooking spray, *Pam* (1¼ second spray)	7	0	1.0	Tr.	0	0
● Vegetable oil spread, *Blue Bonnet* (1 Tbsp.)	80	0	8.0	2.0	0	110
● Vegetable oil spread, *Fleischmann's* (1 Tbsp.)	80	0	8.0	2.0	0	110
● Vegetable oil spread, *Shedd's Nuspread* (1 Tbsp.)	70	0	7.0	1.0	0	110
BUTTER						
● ■ Salted (1 Tbsp.)	102	11.5	0.1	6.3	35	140
● Substitute, *Butter Buds* (2 tsp.)	12	1.0	0	0	0	220
■ Unsalted (1 Tbsp.)	102	0.1	11.5	6.3	35	1
■ Unsalted, *Land O' Lakes* (1 Tbsp.)	100	0	11.0	7.0	31	2

Alerts: ● Sodium ★ Sugar ■ Cholesterol

Food Description	Calories	Carbohydrates (grams)	Fat (grams)	Saturated Fat (grams)	Cholesterol (milligrams)	Sodium (milligrams)
●■ Whipped, *Land O' Lakes* (1 Tbsp.)	100	0	11.0	7.0	31	111
●■ Whipped, lightly salted, *Land O' Lakes* (1 Tbsp.)	60	0	7.0	4.0	20	71
●■ Whipped, salted (1 Tbsp.)	67	0	7.6	4.2	23	93
■ Whipped, unsalted (1 Tbsp.)	67	0	7.6	4.2	23	1
■ Whipped, unsalted, *Land O' Lakes* (1 Tbsp.)	60	0	7.0	4.0	20	1
MARGARINE						
● *Autumn* (1 Tbsp.)	100	0	11.2	2.5	0	NA
● Diet, *Blue Bonnet* (1 Tbsp.)	50	0	6.0	1.0	0	110
● Diet, *Fleischmann's* (1 Tbsp.)	50	0	6.0	NA	0	110
● Diet, *Imperial* (1 Tbsp.)	50	0	6.0	1.2	Tr.	NA
● Diet, *Mazola* (1 Tbsp.)	50	0	6.0	1.0	0	135
● *Fleischmann's* (1 Tbsp.)	100	0	11.0	NA	0	110
● *Imperial* (1 Tbsp.)	100	0	11.2	2.5	Tr.	NA
● *Kraft Parkay* (1 Tbsp.)	100	0	11.0	2.0	0	110
● *Land O' Lakes* (1 Tbsp.)	100	0	11.0	2.0	0	111
● *Mazola* (1 Tbsp.)	100	0	11.0	2.0	0	115
● *Promise* (1 Tbsp.)	100	0	11.2	2.0	0	NA
● Reduced calorie, *Weight Watchers* (1 Tbsp.)	50	0	6.0	1.0	0	111
● Salted (1 Tbsp.)	102	0.1	11.5	2.1	0	140
● Soft, *Autumn* (1 Tbsp.)	100	0	11.2	2.2	0	NA
● Soft, *Blue Bonnet* (1 Tbsp.)	100	0	11.0	2.0	0	110
● Soft, *Chiffon* (1 Tbsp.)	90	0	10.0	2.0	0	105
● Soft, *Fleischmann's* (1 Tbsp.)	100	0	11.0	NA	0	110
● Soft, *Imperial* (1 Tbsp.)	100	0	11.2	2.2	0	NA
● Soft, *Kraft Parkay* (1 Tbsp.)	100	0	11.0	2.0	0	115
● Soft, *Promise* (1 Tbsp.)	100	0	11.2	1.7	0	NA
● Soft, stick, *Chiffon* (1 Tbsp.)	100	0	11.0	2	0	110
Soft, unsalted, *Fleischmann's* (1 Tbsp.)	100	0	11.0	NA	0	10
Soft, unsalted, *Soft Chiffon* (1 Tbsp.)	90	0	10.0	2.0	0	0
● Soft, whipped, *Fleischmann's* (1 Tbsp.)	70	0	7.0	2.0	0	70
Unsalted (1 Tbsp.)	102	0.1	11.5	2.1	0	1
Unsalted, *Fleischmann's* (1 Tbsp.)	100	0	11.0	NA	0	10
Unsalted, *Mazola* (1 Tbsp.)	100	0	11.0	2.0	0	0
● Whipped, *Blue Bonnet* (1 Tbsp.)	70	0	7.0	2.0	0	70
● Whipped, *Imperial* (1 Tbsp.)	65	0	7.0	1.4	0	NA
● Whipped, salted (1 Tbsp.)	68	0	7.6	1.5	0	93

Alerts: ● Sodium ★ Sugar ■ Cholesterol

Food Description	Calories	Carbohydrates (grams)	Fat (grams)	Saturated Fat (grams)	Cholesterol (milligrams)	Sodium (milligrams)
• Whipped, *Soft Chiffon* (1 Tbsp.)	70	0	8.0	1.0	0	80
Whipped, unsalted (1 Tbsp.)	68	0	7.6	1.5	0	1

Fish and Seafood

All fish and seafood contain cholesterol and sodium in varying amounts. If you are restricting either of these two food constituents in your diet, you should maintain an awareness of your cholesterol or sodium intake when you consume fish and seafood. We have assigned an alert to a particular item only when the cholesterol or sodium content may be considered unacceptably high—due to the nature of the food or the method of processing or preparation—when compared to other fish and seafood items.

Food Description	Calories	Carbohydrates (grams)	Fat (grams)	Saturated Fat (grams)	Cholesterol (milligrams)	Sodium (milligrams)
• Anchovies, pickled, canned (5 filets)	35	0.1	2.1	1.0	11	165
• Bass, striped, ovenfried (7 oz. filet)	392	13.4	17.0	6.0	126	NA
Bass, striped, raw (3½ oz.)	105	0	2.7	1.0	55	68
Bass, black sea, stuffed, baked (7 oz. filet)	531	23.4	32.4	10.3	94	139
Bluefish, baked with butter (5.5 oz. filet)	246	0	8.1	1.6	109	161
• Bluefish, fried (7 oz. filet)	400	9.2	19.1	3.9	119	285
Bluefish, raw (3½ oz.)	117	0	3.3	1.0	55	74
Buffalo, raw (3½ oz.)	113	0	4.2	1.0	55	52
• ▪ Burbot, fried (1 lb.)	748	0	29.0	4.5	531	803
Catfish, freshwater, raw (3½ oz.)	103	0	3.1	1.0	55	61
• ▪ Caviar, granular (1 Tbsp.)	42	0.5	2.4	0.5	48	352
Chub, raw (3½ oz.)	145	0	8.8	2.0	55	81
• Clams (4 cherrystones or 5 little necks)	56	4.1	0.6	0	35	144
• Clams, canned, drained, minced (1 cup)	157	3.0	4.0	0	101	192
• Clams, hard shell (1 pint)	363	26.8	4.1	0	227	930
• Clams, light batter fried, frozen, *Mrs. Paul's* (2½ oz.)	270	25.0	16.0	NA	NA	675
• Clam liquor, canned (1 oz.)	6.0	0.6	0	0	3	120

Alerts: • Sodium ★ Sugar ▪ Cholesterol

Food Description	Calories	Carbohydrates (grams)	Fat (grams)	Saturated Fat (grams)	Cholesterol (milligrams)	Sodium (milligrams)
Clams, soft shell (1 pint)	372	5.9	8.6	0	227	163
• Clams, with liquid, canned (7½-8 oz.)	114	6.2	1.5	0	70	1254
• Cod, broiled with butter (2.3 oz. filet)	110	0	3.4	0.7	53	71
• Cod, broiled with butter (8.3 oz steak)	352	0	11.0	2.1	168	228
• Cod, flaked, canned, drained (4½ oz.)	204	0	0.7	0	132	264
• Cod, dehydrated, lightly salted (1 oz.)	106	0	0.8	0	66	2296
Cod, raw (3½ oz.)	78	0	0.3	0	50	70
• Crab, claw meat, canned, drained (1 cup)	116	1.3	2.9	0	116	1150
• Crab, king, canned, *Pacific Pearl* (6½ oz.)	100	1.7	1.7	0	82	810
• Crabmeat, Alaska King, cooked, frozen, *Wakefield* (3 oz.)	60	1.0	1.0	0	49	400
• Crabmeat, Alaska Snow, cooked, frozen, *Wakefield* (3 oz.)	60	1.0	1.0	0	49	400
• Crab, miniatures, deviled, frozen, *Mrs. Paul's* (3½ oz.)	210	24.0	9.0	NA	NA	700
• Crab, snow, canned, *Pacific Pearl* (6½ oz.)	100	1.7	1.7	0	82	895
• Crab, steamed, flaked (1 cup)	116	0.6	2.4	0	125	262
• Crab, steamed (3½ oz.)	93	0.5	1.9	0	100	210
• Cusk, steamed (1 lb.)	481	0	3.2	0	340	335
• Fish cakes, thin, frozen, *Mrs. Paul's* (5 oz.)	320	31.0	18.0	NA	NA	1850
• Fishcakes, frozen, fried (1 lb.)	1225	78.0	81.2	31.8	118	802
•■ Fish filets, buttered, frozen, *Mrs. Paul's* (2 filets)	310	2.0	26.0	NA	NA	600
• Fish filets, supreme-light batter fried, frozen, *Mrs. Paul's* (3⅝ oz.)	220	19.0	10.0	NA	NA	508
• Fish sticks, frozen, *Booth* (4 oz.)	220	25.0	8.0	NA	NA	NA
• Fish stick, frozen (1 oz.)	50	1.8	2.5	0.9	13	50
• Fish sticks, frozen, *Mrs. Paul's* (4 sticks)	150	16.0	5.0	NA	NA	540
• Flounder, baked with butter (1 large filet)	202	0	8.2	2.0	90	237
• Flounder, filets, fried, frozen, *Mrs. Paul's* (4 oz.)	220	22.0	10.0	NA	NA	760

Alerts: • Sodium ★ Sugar ■ Cholesterol

Food Description	Calories	Carbohydrates (grams)	Fat (grams)	Saturated Fat (grams)	Cholesterol (milligrams)	Sodium (milligrams)
• Flounder, lemon butter, frozen, *Mrs. Paul's* (4¼ oz.)	150	9.0	8.0	NA	NA	808
Flounder, raw (3½ oz.)	79	0	0.8	0	50	78
Grouper, raw (3½ oz.)	87	0	0.5	0	55	61
• Haddock, filets, fried, frozen, *Mrs. Paul's* (4 oz.)	230	24.0	9.0	NA	NA	1120
• Haddock, fried (4 oz. filet)	181	6.4	7.0	1.1	70	195
Haddock, raw (3½ oz.)	79	0	0.1	0	60	61
Hake, raw (3½ oz.)	74	0	0.4	0	55	74
Halibut, Atlantic and Pacific, raw (3½ oz.)	100	0	1.2	0	50	54
• Halibut, broiled with butter (4.4 oz. filet)	214	0	8.7	2.5	75	168
Herring, Atlantic, raw (3½ oz.)	176	0	11.3	2.0	85	74
• Herring, pickled, pieces (½ oz.)	33	0	2.3	0.4	15	935
• Herring, smoked, kippered, canned, drained (1 medium filet)	84	0	5.2	1.0	44	2492
• Lobster, canned or cooked, pieces (1 cup)	138	0.4	2.2	0	123	305
• Lobster, northern, cooked (3½ oz.)	95	0.3	1.5	0	85	210
Mackerel, Atlantic, broiled with butter (3.7 oz. filet)	248	0	16.6	5.3	106	78
Mackerel, Atlantic, raw (3½ oz.)	191	0	12.2	4.0	95	74
• Mackerel, salted (4 oz. filet)	342	0	28.1	9.0	106	6978
• Mussels, Atlantic and Pacific, meat and liquid, raw (3½ oz.)	66	3.1	1.4	0	50	289
• Oysters, frozen (12 oz.)	274	17.6	7.9	0	162	1368
• Oysters, fried (4 medium or 1.6 oz.)	108	8.4	6.3	0.9	20	93
• Oysters, boiled, canned, *Pacific Pearl* (8 oz.)	170	11	5	0	77	850
• Oysters, raw, Eastern, chilled (1 cup)	158	8.2	4.3	0	120	175
• Oysters, raw, Pacific/Western, chilled (1 cup)	218	15.4	5.3	0	120	175
• Oysters, shelled, canned, *Bumble Bee* (1 cup)	218	15.4	5.3	0	NA	185
Perch, Atlantic, raw (3½ oz.)	88	0	1.2	0	55	79
• Perch, filets, ocean, frozen, *Mrs. Paul's* (4 oz.)	250	18.0	14.0	NA	NA	800

Alerts: • Sodium ★ Sugar ■ Cholesterol

Food Description	Calories	Carbohydrates (grams)	Fat (grams)	Saturated Fat (grams)	Cholesterol (milligrams)	Sodium (milligrams)
● Perch, ocean, frozen, breaded, fried, reheated (3.2 oz filet)	281	14.5	16.6	2.6	51	135
Perch, yellow, raw (3½ oz.)	91	0	0.9	0	55	68
Pickerel, chain, raw (3½ oz.)	84	0	0.5	0	55	68
Pike, northern, raw (3½ oz.)	88	0	1.1	0	55	51
Pike, walleye, raw (3 oz.)	93	0	1.2	0	55	51
● Pollock, cooked, creamed (1 cup)	320	10.0	14.8	7.5	93	278
Rockfish, raw (3½ oz.)	97	0	1.8	0	55	60
Rockfish, steamed (4 oz. filet)	123	2.2	2.9	0	61	78
● Salmon, broiled with butter (5 oz. steak)	232	0	9.4	2.6	60	148
Salmon, coho, raw (3½ oz.)	186	0	10.9	3.0	33	48
● Salmon, keta, canned, salted, *Bumble Bee* (1 cup)	306	0	11.4	NA	NA	NA
Salmon, low sodium, canned, *Nutradiet* (½ cup)	188	0	11.0	NA	NA	45
● Salmon, pink, canned, *Del Monte* (7¾ oz.)	310	0	13.0	NA	NA	1220
● Salmon, pink, canned, no salt, *Featherweight* (3⅞ oz.)	NA	NA	NA	NA	NA	95
● Salmon, pink, canned, salted, *Bumble Bee* (1 cup)	310	0	13.0	NA	NA	851
● Salmon, pink/humpback, canned, with salt (7¾ oz.)	310	0	13.0	3.4	77	851
● Salmon, red sockeye, canned, *Del Monte* (7¾ oz.)	340	0	17.0	NA	NA	1170
● Salmon, red sockeye, canned, salted, *Bumble Bee* (1 cup)	376	0	20.5	NA	NA	1148
● Salmon, red sockeye, canned with salt (7¾ oz.)	376	0	20.5	6.6	77	1148
Salmon, sockeye, raw (3½ oz.)	186	0	10.9	3.0	35	48
● Salmon, smoked (1 oz.)	50	0	2.6	0.9	11	1767
● Sardines, Atlantic, canned in oil, drained (3½ oz.)	203	0	11.1	2.0	140	823
● Sardines, canned, drained (1 medium)	24	0	1.3	0.2	17	99
● Sardines, canned, water pack, *Featherweight* (1⅞ oz.)	NA	NA	NA	NA	NA	65
● Sardines, canned in oil (3¾ oz.)	330	0.6	25.9	5.3	127	541
● Sardines, canned in oil, *Crown Norway* (3 oz.)	260	1.0	20	NA	NA	NA

Alerts: ● Sodium ★ Sugar ■ Cholesterol

Food Description	Calories	Carbohydrates (grams)	Fat (grams)	Saturated Fat (grams)	Cholesterol (milligrams)	Sodium (milligrams)
•★ Sardines, canned, in tomato sauce, *Del Monte* (7½ oz.)	330	4.0	18.0	NA	NA	825
• Sardines, chunk light, *Pacific Pearl* (7 oz.)	250	NA	6.0	NA	105	780
• Sardines, in mustard sauce, *King Oscar* (3¾ oz.)	240	2.0	18.0	NA	NA	NA
• Sardines, in olive oil, *King Oscar* (3¾ oz.)	260	1.0	20.0	NA	NA	NA
• Sardines, Norway brisling, canned in soya oil, *King Oscar* (3¾ oz.)	260	1.0	20.0	NA	NA	NA
• Sardines, Norway brisling, canned in tomato sauce, *King Oscar* (3¾ oz.)	240	2.0	18.0	NA	NA	NA
• Scallops, bay and sea, raw (3½ oz.)	81	3.3	0.2	0	35	255
• Scallops, breaded, fried, frozen, reheated (6⅔ oz./yield of 7 oz. package)	367	19.8	15.9	3.8	77	227
• Scallops, light batter, frozen, *Mrs. Paul's* (3½ oz.)	200	21.0	8.0	NA	NA	735
• Scallops, steamed (1 lb.)	508	15.0	6.4	0	240	1202
• Seafood platter, frozen, *Mrs. Paul's* (9 oz.)	510	57.0	22.0	NA	NA	2160
Shad, baked (1 oz.)	57	0	3.2	1.1	20	22
Shad, raw (3½ oz.)	170	0	10.0	3.0	55	54
•■ Shrimp, Alaska, cooked, frozen, *Wakefield* (3 oz.)	66	2.0	1.0	0	136	468
•■ Shrimp, canned (10 large)	67	0.4	0.6	0	87	81
•■ Shrimp, canned (10 medium)	37	0.2	0.4	0	48	45
•■ Shrimp, canned, *Pacific Pearl* (4¼ oz.)	94	3	1.4	0	193	980
•■ Shrimp, cooked, frozen, *Brilliant* (6 oz.)	100	0	2.0	0	NA	NA
•■ Shrimp, French fried (1 lb.)	1021	45.4	49.0	9.1	680	844
•■ Shrimp, fried, frozen, *Mrs. Paul's* (3 oz.)	170	17.0	11.0	NA	NA	480
•■ Shrimp paste, canned (1 tsp.)	13	0.1	0.7	0.4	12	10
•■ Shrimp, raw (3½ oz.)	91	1.5	0.8	0	150	140
Smelt, raw (3½ oz.)	98	0	2.1	1.0	55	70
Snails, raw (3½ oz.)	90	2.0	1.4	0	50	70
Snapper, red and grey, raw (3½ oz.)	93	0	0.9	0	55	67
• Snow crabmeat and shrimp, *Pacific Pearl* (3 oz.)	60	1.0	1.0	0	49	400

Alerts: • Sodium ★ Sugar ■ Cholesterol

Food Description	Calories	Carbohydrates (grams)	Fat (grams)	Saturated Fat (grams)	Cholesterol (milligrams)	Sodium (milligrams)
• Sole, lemon butter, frozen, *Mrs. Paul's* (4¼ oz.)	160	10.0	8.0	NA	NA	808
Sturgeon, raw (3½ oz.)	94	0	1.9	0	55	54
• Sturgeon, smoked (1 oz.)	42	0	0.5	0	27	1767
Sturgeon, steamed (1 oz.)	45	0	1.6	0.6	22	31
• Swordfish, broiled with butter (5 oz. piece)	237	0	8.2	2.7	109	183
Swordfish, raw (3½ oz.)	118	0	4.0	1.0	55	54
Trout, brook, raw (3½ oz.)	101	0	2.1	1.0	49	47
Trout, lake, raw (3½ oz.)	168	0	10.0	3.0	55	81
• Tuna, albacore, canned in oil, *Chicken of the Sea* (3½ oz.)	250	0	17.2	NA	23	600
Tuna, albacore, low sodium, canned in water, *Chicken of the Sea* (3½ oz.)	114	0	1.9	0	35	40
Tuna, canned in water, with no salt, with liquid, solid pack (3½ oz.)	126	0	0.8	0	62	41
• Tuna, canned in oil, with liquid, solid pack (7 oz.)	570	0	40.6	7.5	109	1584
• Tuna, canned in water, with salt, with liquid, solid pack (7 oz.)	251	0	1.6	0	125	1733
• Tuna, canned in oil, solid pack, drained (6 oz.)	333	0	13.9	3.7	110	1352
Tuna, chunk albacore, low sodium, canned in water, drained, *Chicken of the Sea* (3½ oz.)	125	0	1.9	0	35	39
• Tuna, chunk light, canned in oil, *Bumble Bee* (6½ oz.)	460	0	28.0	NA	NA	NA
• Tuna, chunk light, canned in oil, *Del Monte* (6½ oz.)	450	0	29.0	NA	NA	930
• Tuna, chunk light, canned in oil, drained, *Bumble Bee* (5½ oz.)	309	0	12.9	NA	NA	NA
• Tuna, chunk light, canned in oil, *Star-Kist* (6½ oz.)	450	0	30.0	NA	NA	NA
Tuna, chunk light, canned in water, no salt, *Featherweight* (6½ oz.)	210	0	3.0	0	NA	95
• Tuna, light, canned in oil, *Chicken of the Sea* (3½ oz.)	236	0	15.7	NA	30	520
• Tuna, light, canned in water, *Bumble Bee* (6½ oz.)	234	0	1.5	0	NA	NA

Alerts: • Sodium ★ Sugar ■ Cholesterol

Food Description	Calories	Carbohydrates (grams)	Fat (grams)	Saturated Fat (grams)	Cholesterol (milligrams)	Sodium (milligrams)
• Tuna, light, canned in water, drained, *Chicken of the Sea* (3½ oz.)	111	0	0.9	0	60	405
• Tuna, light solid, canned in water, *Star-Kist* (7 oz.)	220	0	3.0	0	NA	NA
• Tuna, solid albacore, canned in water, drained, *Chicken of the Sea* (3½ oz.)	129	0	1.9	0	35	470
• Tuna, solid white, canned in water, *Bumble Bee* (7 oz.)	251	0	1.6	0	NA	NA
• Weakfish, broiled with butter (1 lb.)	943	0	51.7	18.1	372	2540
Weakfish, raw (3½ oz.)	121	0	5.6	2.0	55	75
Whitefish, lake, raw (3½ oz.)	155	0	8.2	3.0	55	52
• Whitefish, smoked (1 oz.)	44	0	2.1	0.6	17	1766

Flours, Meals, and Grains

Food Description	Calories	Carbohydrates (grams)	Fat (grams)	Saturated Fat (grams)	Cholesterol (milligrams)	Sodium (milligrams)
Barley, pearled (1 cup)	696	154.4	2.2	0	0	8
Barley, Scotch, pearled, *Quaker* (¼ cup)	170	36.3	0.5	Tr.	0	4
Bulgur, from hard red winter wheat (1 cup)	602	128.7	2.5	0	0	6
• Bulgur, canned, from hard red winter wheat, seasoned (1 cup)	246	44.3	4.5	1.4	0	621
Bulgur, from white wheat (1 cup)	553	121.1	1.9	0	0	6
Corn meal, degerminated (1 cup)	502	108.2	1.7	0	0	1
Corn meal, degerminated, cooked without salt (1 cup)	120	25.7	0.5	0	0	0
Corn meal, degerminated, white or yellow, *Quaker* (1 oz.)	102	22.2	0.5	0	0	1
Corn meal, degerminated, *Your Choice* (1 oz.)	100	22.0	1.0	Tr.	0	Tr.

Alerts: ● Sodium ★ Sugar ■ Cholesterol

Food Description	Calories	Carbohydrates (grams)	Fat (grams)	Saturated Fat (grams)	Cholesterol (milligrams)	Sodium (milligrams)
• Corn meal mix, self-rising, degerminated, white, *Aunt Jemima* (1 oz.)	99	20.8	0.7	0	0	328
Corn meal, white, *Albers* (1 oz.)	100	22.0	0	0	0	NA
Corn meal, whole ground (1 cup)	433	89.9	4.8	0.5	0	1
Corn starch, *Argo* (1 Tbsp.)	35	8.3	Tr.	0	0	5
Cracker meal, *Nabisco* (1 cup)	440	95.0	1.0	NA	0	NA
• Grits product with imitation ham bits, instant, *Quaker* (1 oz.)	99	21.3	0.3	Tr.	0	658
• Hominy, golden, *Van Camp's* (1 cup)	120	28.0	1.0	Tr.	0	730
• Hominy grits, quick, *Albers* (1 oz.)	150	33.0	0	0	0	NA
• Hominy grits, white, regular or quick, *Aunt Jemima* (1 oz.)	101	22.4	0.2	0	0	101
• Hominy grits, white, regular or quick, *Quaker* (3 Tbsp.)	101	22.4	0.2	0	0	101
FLOURS						
Buckwheat, dark, sifted (1 cup)	326	70.6	2.4	0	0	2
Buckwheat, light, sifted (1 cup)	340	77.9	1.2	0	0	2
Carob (1 cup)	252	113.0	2.0	0	0	0
Corn (1 cup)	431	89.9	3.0	0.3	0	1
Rye, dark (1 cup)	419	87.2	3.3	0	0	1
Rye, light, sifted (1 cup)	364	79.5	1.0	0	0	1
Rye, medium, *Pillsbury* (1 cup)	420	89.0	3.0	0	0	5
Rye/wheat flour, Bohemian style, *Pillsbury's Best* (4 oz.)	400	86.0	1.0	0	0	5
Soybean, defatted (1 lb.)	1479	172.8	4.1	0	0	4
Soybean, *Featherweight* (1 cup)	470	33.0	16.0	NA	0	NA
Soybean, full fat (1 lb.)	1910	137.9	92.1	13.8	0	4
White Wheat						
All-purpose, *Pillsbury* (1 cup)	400	87.0	1.0	0	0	5
Bread, high protein, high gluten, *Pillsbury's Best* (4 oz.)	410	86.0	1.0	0	0	5
Bread, unsifted, dipped (1 cup)	500	102.3	1.5	0	0	3

Alerts: • Sodium ★ Sugar ■ Cholesterol

Food Description	Calories	Carbohydrates (grams)	Fat (grams)	Saturated Fat (grams)	Cholesterol (milligrams)	Sodium (milligrams)
Cake, bleached, *Swans Down* (¼ cup)	100	22.0	0	0	0	NA
Cake or pastry, sifted, spooned (1 cup)	349	76.2	0.8	0	0	2
Gluten, *Featherweight* (1 cup)	420	55.0	2.0	0	0	NA
Gluten, spooned (1 cup)	510	63.7	2.6	0	0	3
High protein, *Gold Medal* (4 oz.)	400	83.0	1.0	0	0	5
•Self-rising, *Gold Medal* (4 oz.)	380	83.0	1.0	0	0	1520
•Self-rising, sifted, spooned (1 cup)	405	85.3	1.1	0	0	1240
•Self-rising, unsifted, spooned (1 cup)	440	92.8	1.3	0	0	1348
Wheat, all-purpose, bleached, pre-sifted, *Gold Medal* (4 oz.)	400	87.0	1.0	0	0	5
Wheat, all-purpose, unbleached, pre-sifted *Ceresota* (4 oz.)	400	85.0	1.0	0	0	0
Wheat, all-purpose, unbleached, pre-sifted, *Gold Medal* (1 cup)	400	87.0	1.0	0	0	5
Wheat, all-purpose, unbleached, pre-sifted, *Pillsbury's Best* (4 oz.)	400	86.0	1.0	0	0	5
Wheat, bleached, instant blending, spooned (1 cup)	470	98.2	1.3	0	0	3
Wheat, bleached, instant mixing, *Wondra* (1 cup)	400	87.0	1.0	0	0	5
Wheat, bleached, unsifted, dipped (1 cup)	499	104.3	1.4	0	0	3
•Wheat, self-rising, *Aunt Jemima* (1 oz.)	100	21.0	0	0	0	NA
Wheat, tortilla, *Azteca* (0.9 oz.)	78	14.6	1.2	0	0	81
Whole wheat, graham, *Pillsbury's Best* (4 oz.)	400	80.0	2.0	0	0	10
Whole wheat, unbleached, crushed, *Ceresota* (1 cup)	400	80.0	2.0	0	0	0
RICE AND RICE DISHES						
Brown, dry, *Riceland* (2¾ oz.)	280	60.3	1.5	0	0	7
Brown, dry, *Uncle Ben's* (3½ oz.)	370	74.5	4.2	0	0	13
•Brown, prepared with salt, hot (1 cup)	232	49.7	1.2	0	0	549

Alerts: •Sodium ★Sugar ■Cholesterol

Food Description	Calories	Carbohydrates (grams)	Fat (grams)	Saturated Fat (grams)	Cholesterol (milligrams)	Sodium (milligrams)
• Brown/wild, dry, seasoned, *Uncle Ben's* (3½ oz.)	362	25	4.2	0	0	1360
• Continental (green beans, almonds), frozen, *Green Giant Boil-in-Bag* (3½ oz.)	88	13.7	3.0	NA	NA	432
Converted long grain, dry, *Uncle Ben's* (3½ oz.)	355	79.3	0.6	0	0	5
Enriched, long grain, prepared without salt, hot (1 cup)	185	40.8	0.2	0	0	0
• Enriched, long grain, prepared with salt, cold (1 cup)	154	33.8	0.1	0	0	519
• French style, frozen, *Birds Eye International Recipe* (3.6 oz.)	110	23.0	0	0	NA	750
• Fried, chicken, prepared, *La Choy* (½ cup)	209	40.1	1.9	0.6	8	1153
• Fried, Chinese style, prepared, *La Choy* (½ cup)	207	42.8	1.9	0.4	1	1225
Instant, prepared without salt, hot (1 cup)	180	39.9	0	0	0	0
Long grain, dry, *Riceland* (2¾ oz.)	283	62.7	0.3	0	0	4
• Long grain/wild, dry, *Minute Rice* (½ cup)	120	25.0	0	0	0	535
• Long grain/wild, dry, seasoned, *Uncle Ben's* (3½ oz.)	343	72.5	1.0	0	0	1480
• Mix, dry, chicken flavor, *Rice-A-Roni* (1.6 oz.)	160	33.0	1.0	NA	NA	NA
• Mix, dry, drumstick flavor, *Minute Rice* (to make 1 serving)	120	25.0	0	0	0	460
Mix, dry, *Minute Rice* (to make ⅔ cup)	120	25.0	0	0	0	0
• Mix, dry, rib roast flavor, *Minute Rice* (to make 1 serving)	120	25.0	0	0	0	550
• Oriental style, frozen, *Birds Eye International Recipe* (3.6 oz.)	130	27.0	1.0	NA	NA	655
• Pilaf/mushrooms/onions, frozen, *Green Giant* (1 cup)	230	45.0	4.0	NA	NA	533
Spanish, canned, *Featherweight* (7½ oz.)	140	30.0	0	0	0	32
• Spanish, canned, *Van Camp's* (1 cup)	190	31.0	5.0	NA	NA	1480

Alerts: • Sodium ★ Sugar ■ Cholesterol

Food Description	Calories	Carbohydrates (grams)	Fat (grams)	Saturated Fat (grams)	Cholesterol (milligrams)	Sodium (milligrams)
• Spanish style, frozen, *Birds Eye* (3.6 oz.)	100	20.0	0	0	NA	785
• Verdi (bell peppers, parsley), *Green Giant Boil-in-Bag* (3½ oz.)	108	20.5	2.5	NA	NA	480
• White/wild, frozen, *Green Giant Boil-in-Bag* (3½ oz.)	91	18.8	0.8	0	0	461
Wild, dry (1 cup)	565	120.5	1.1	0	0	11

Fruits

	Calories	Carbohydrates (grams)	Fat (grams)	Saturated Fat (grams)	Cholesterol (milligrams)	Sodium (milligrams)
Apple (1 medium)	80	20.0	0.8	0	0	1
• Apple fritters, frozen, *Mrs. Paul* (2 fritters)	240	32.0	12.0	NA	NA	1080
Applesauce						
★ Canned, *Del Monte* (1 cup)	170	47.0	0	0	0	10
★ Canned, *Musselman* (1 cup)	193	47.0	0.4	NA	0	NA
Canned, natural, *Musselman* (1 cup)	100	24.0	0	0	0	NA
Canned, *Nutradiet* (½ cup)	55	14.0	0	0	0	NA
★ Canned, *S & W* (1 cup)	170	47.0	0	NA	NA	NA
★ Canned, *Stokely-Van Camp* (1 cup)	180	46.0	0	0	0	70
★ Canned, sweetened (1 cup)	232	60.7	0.3	0	0	5
★ Canned, sweetened, *Mott's* (8 oz.)	230	55.0	0	0	0	10
Canned, unsweetened (1 cup)	100	26.4	0.5	0	0	5
Canned, unsweetened, *Featherweight* (½ cup)	50	12.0	0	0	0	10
Canned, unsweetened, *Seneca* (½ cup)	50	12.0	0	0	0	10
★ With cranberries, canned, *Mott's* (8 oz.)	220	54.0	0	0	0	10
Apples, dehydrated (1 cup)	353	92.1	2.0	0	0	7
★ Apples, dried, rings, prepared with sugar (1 cup)	314	81.8	1.1	0	0	3
• Apples, dry, *Del Monte* (2 oz.)	140	37.0	0	0	0	60

Alerts: • Sodium ★ Sugar ■ Cholesterol

Food Description	Calories	Carbohydrates (grams)	Fat (grams)	Saturated Fat (grams)	Cholesterol (milligrams)	Sodium (milligrams)
•★Apples, frozen, sliced, sweetened (1 lb.)	422	110.2	0.5	0	0	299
Apples, pared, sliced or diced (1 cup)	59	15.5	0.3	0	0	1
★Apricot filling, *Solo* (1 oz.)	48	11.8	Tr.	0	0	7
Apricots						
Apricots (3)	55	13.7	0.2	0	0	1
★Canned, extra light syrup, halves, *Del Monte Lite* (1 cup)	120	30.0	0	0	0	NA
★Canned, grape juice pack, halves, *Diet Delight* (½ cup)	60	15.0	0	0	0	12
★Canned, heavy syrup, halves with liquid (1 cup)	222	56.8	0.3	0	0	3
Canned in juice, halves, *Nutradiet* (½ cup)	50	13.0	0	0	0	NA
Canned in water, *Featherweight* (½ cup)	35	9.0	0	0	0	10
Canned in water, halves, *Nutradiet* (½ cup)	35	9.0	0	0	0	NA
Canned, juice pack, halves, *Featherweight* (½ cup)	50	12.0	0	0	0	10
★Canned, *Stokely-Van Camp* (1 cup)	220	54.0	0	0	0	45
Canned, water pack, halves, with liquid (1 cup)	93	23.6	0.2	0	0	2
★Canned, whole, peeled, *Del Monte* (1 cup)	200	53.0	0	0	0	40
Dried, halves (1 cup)	338	86.4	0.6	0	0	33
Dry, *Del Monte* (2 oz.)	140	35.0	0	0	0	10
★Frozen, sweetened (8 oz.)	227	55.7	0.2	NA	0	9
Avocado (½)	188	7.1	18.4	3.7	0	4
Avocados, cubed (1 cup)	251	9.4	24.6	4.9	0	6
Avocados, pureed (1 cup)	384	14.5	37.7	7.5	0	9
Banana (1 medium)	101	26.4	0.2	0	0	1
Bananas, dehydrated, flakes (1 oz.)	96	25.1	0.2	0	0	1
Bananas, mashed (1 cup)	191	49.9	0.4	0	0	2
Bananas, red, sliced (1 cup)	135	35.1	0.3	0	0	1
★Blackberries, canned, heavy syrup (1 cup)	233	56.8	1.5	0	0	3
Blackberries, canned, water pack (1 cup)	98	22.0	1.5	0	0	2
Blackberries/dewberries/ boysenberries/youngberries (1 cup)	84	18.6	1.3	0	0	1

Alerts: • Sodium ★ Sugar ■ Cholesterol

Food Description	Calories	Carbohydrates (grams)	Fat (grams)	Saturated Fat (grams)	Cholesterol (milligrams)	Sodium (milligrams)
Blueberries (1 cup)	90	22.2	0.7	0	0	1
★Blueberries, frozen, sweetened (1 cup)	241	60.9	0.7	0	0	2
Blueberries, frozen, unsweetened (1 cup)	91	22.4	0.8	0	0	2
★Blueberry filling, *Solo* (1 oz.)	53	13.2	Tr.	0	0	7
Boysenberries, canned, water pack, with liquid (1 cup)	163	41.3	0.5	0	0	4
★Boysenberries, frozen, sweetened (1 cup)	137	34.9	0.4	0	0	1
Boysenberries, frozen, unsweetened (1 cup)	60	14.4	0.4	0	0	1
Cantaloupe (5″ melon)	159	39.7	0.5	0	0	63
Cantaloupe balls (1 cup)	48	12.0	0.2	0	0	19
Casaba (6½″ melon)	367	88.5	0	0	0	163
Casaba melon balls (1 cup)	46	11.0	0	0	0	20
Cherries						
Dark sweet, canned in water, *Featherweight* (½ cup)	60	13.0	0	0	0	10
★Dark sweet, canned, pitted, *Del Monte* (1 cup)	190	50.0	1.0	NA	0	10
★Light sweet, canned, *Del Monte* (1 cup)	190	51.0	0	0	0	10
Light sweet, canned in water, *Featherweight* (½ cup)	50	11.0	0	0	0	10
Red, sour, canned, pitted, *Stokely-Van Camp* (1 cup)	90	21.0	0	0	0	40
Sour (1 lb.)	237	58.4	1.2	0	0	8
Sour, canned, water pack, pitted (1 cup)	105	26.1	0.5	0	0	5
★Sour, frozen, sweetened (1 lb.)	508	126.1	1.8	0	0	9
Sour, pitted (1 cup)	90	22.2	0.5	0	0	3
Sweet (1 lb.)	286	71.0	1.2	0	0	8
★Sweet, canned, heavy syrup, pitted (1 cup)	208	52.7	0.5	0	0	3
★Sweet, canned in heavy syrup, whole, *Libby* (1 cup)	200	53.0	0	0	0	10
Sweet, canned, water pack (1 cup)	119	29.6	0.5	0	0	2
Sweet, pitted (1 cup)	102	25.2	0.4	0	0	3
★Cherry filling, *Solo* (1 oz.)	84	21.1	0	0	0	7
Cranberries (1 cup)	44	10.3	0.7	0	0	2
★Cranberry-orange relish (1 cup)	489	124.8	1.1	0	0	3

Alerts: ● Sodium ★ Sugar ■ Cholesterol

Food Description	Calories	Carbohydrates (grams)	Fat (grams)	Saturated Fat (grams)	Cholesterol (milligrams)	Sodium (milligrams)
★Cranberry sauce, canned, jelly, *Ocean Spray* (2 oz.)	90	22.0	0	0	0	17
★Cranberry sauce, canned, whole, *Ocean Spray* (2 oz.)	90	22.0	0	0	0	16
★Cranberry sauce, sweetened, homemade, unstrained (1 cup)	493	126.0	0.8	0	0	3
★Cran-orange relish, frozen, *Ocean Spray* (2 oz.)	100	26.0	0	0	0	18
★Currants, zonte, canned, *Del Monte* (½ cup)	190	48.0	0	0	0	10
●★Date filling, *Solo* (1 oz.)	64	15.3	0.2	NA	0	25
Dates (8 oz.)	541	143.9	1.0	0	0	2
Dates (10 fruits)	219	58.3	0.4	0	0	Tr.
Dates, chopped (1 cup)	488	129.8	0.9	0	0	2
Dates, chopped, *Dromedary* (¼ cup)	130	31.0	0	0	0	NA
Dates, pitted, *Dromedary* (5)	100	23.0	0	0	0	NA
Fig (1 medium)	40	10.1	0.1	0	0	1
★Figs, canned, heavy syrup, with liquid (1 cup)	218	56.5	0.5	0	0	5
Figs, canned, water pack, with liquid (1 cup)	119	30.8	0.5	0	0	5
Figs, kadota, canned in water, *Featherweight* (½ cup)	60	15.0	0	0	0	10
★Figs, whole, canned, *Del Monte* (1 cup)	210	55.0	0	0	0	10
Fruit Cocktail						
★Canned, extra light syrup, *Del Monte Lite* (1 cup)	110	28.0	0	0	0	NA
★Canned, grape juice pack, *Diet Delight* (½ cup)	50	14.0	0	0	0	12
★Canned, heavy syrup, *Libby* (1 cup)	170	45.0	0	0	0	20
★Canned, heavy syrup, with liquid (1 cup)	194	50.2	0.3	0	0	12
Canned in juice, *Featherweight* (½ cup)	50	12.0	0	0	0	10
Canned in juice, *Libby* (1 cup)	150	40.0	0	0	0	10
Canned in water, *Featherweight* (½ cup)	40	10.0	0	0	0	10
Canned in water, *Nutradiet* (½ cup)	40	10.0	0	0	0	NA
Canned, juice pack, *Libby Lite* (½ cup)	50	13.0	0	0	0	10

Alerts: ● Sodium ★ Sugar ■ Cholesterol

Food Description	Calories	Carbohydrates (grams)	Fat (grams)	Saturated Fat (grams)	Cholesterol (milligrams)	Sodium (milligrams)
★Canned, *Stokely-Van Camp* (1 cup)	190	46.0	0	0	0	30
★Canned, water pack, *Diet Delight* (½ cup)	40	10.0	0	0	0	12
★Canned, water pack, with liquid (1 cup)	91	23.8	0.2	0	0	12
Fruit salad, canned, *Diet Delight* (½ cup)	60	16.0	0	0	0	12
★Fruit salad, canned, heavy syrup, *Del Monte* (1 cup)	170	46.0	0	0	0	10
Fruit salad, canned in juice, *Nutradiet* (½ cup)	60	14.0	0	0	0	NA
Fruit salad, canned in water, *Featherweight* (½ cup)	40	10.0	0	0	0	10
Fruit salad, canned in water, *Nutradiet* (½ cup)	35	10.0	0	0	0	NA
Fruit salad, canned, juice pack, *Featherweight* (½ cup)	50	12.0	0	0	0	10
★Fruit salad, canned, *Stokely-Van Camp* (1 cup)	190	44.0	1.0	NA	0	30
Gooseberries (1 cup)	59	14.6	0.3	0	0	2
Granadilla, purple — passion fruit (1)	16	3.9	0.1	0	0	5
Grapefruit						
Canned in juice, sections, *Del Monte* (1 cup)	90	21.0	0	0	0	10
Canned in juice, sections, *Nutradiet* (½ cup)	40	9.0	0	0	0	NA
★Canned in syrup, sections, *Del Monte* (1 cup)	140	35.0	0	0	0	10
Canned, juice pack, segments, *Featherweight* (½ cup)	40	9.0	0	0	0	10
★Canned, *Kraft* (½ cup)	60	14.0	0	0	0	NA
Canned, water pack, sections, with liquid (1 cup)	73	18.5	0.2	0	0	9
Pink and red (½ medium)	58	15.0	0.1	0	0	1
Pink and red, seedless (½ medium)	49	12.8	0.1	0	0	1
Sections (1 cup)	82	21.2	0.2	0	0	2
Sections with juice (1 cup)	94	24.4	0.2	0	0	2
White (½ medium)	56	14.7	0.1	0	0	1
White, seedless (½ medium)	46	11.9	0.1	0	0	1
Grapes, American (1 cup)	70	15.9	1.0	0	0	3

Alerts: ● Sodium ★ Sugar ■ Cholesterol

Food Description	Calories	Carbohydrates (grams)	Fat (grams)	Saturated Fat (grams)	Cholesterol (milligrams)	Sodium (milligrams)
Grapes, American—Concord, Delaware, Niagara, Catawba, Scuppernong (8 oz.)	104	23.5	1.5	0	0	5
★Grapes, canned, Thompson seedless, heavy syrup (1 cup)	197	51.2	0.3	0	0	10
Grapes, canned, Thompson seedless, water pack, with liquid (1 cup)	125	33.3	0.2	0	0	9
Grapes, European, seedless (1 cup)	107	27.7	0.5	0	0	5
Grapes, European—Thompson Seedless, Emperor, Flame Tokay, Ribier, Malaga, Muscat (8 oz.)	152	39.3	0.7	0	0	7
Grapes, seedless, canned in water, *Featherweight* (½ cup)	60	13.0	0	0	0	10
Honeydew (7″ melon)	495	115.5	4.5	0	0	179
Honeydew melon balls (1 cup)	56	13.1	0.5	0	0	20
Kumquat (1 medium)	12	3.2	0	0	0	1
Lemon (1 large)	29	8.7	0.3	0	0	2
Lemon (1 wedge)	7	2.2	0.1	0	0	Tr.
Lime (1)	19	6.4	0.1	0	0	1
Loganberries (1 lb.)	281	67.6	2.7	0	0	4
Loquats (10)	59	15.3	0.2	0	0	2
Mango (1)	152	38.8	0.9	0	0	16
Mangos, diced or sliced (1 cup)	109	27.7	0.7	0	0	11
★Mixed fruit, canned, extra light syrup, chunks, *Del Monte Lite* (1 cup)	100	25.0	0	0	0	NA
★Mixed fruit, canned, heavy syrup, chunks, *Libby* (1 cup)	190	50.0	0	0	0	15
Mixed fruit, canned, juice pack, chunks, *Libby Lite* (½ cup)	50	13.0	0	0	0	10
★Mixed fruit cup, canned, *Del Monte* (5 oz.)	100	27.0	0	0	0	10
★Mixed fruit, frozen, Quick Thaw Pouch, *Birds Eye* (5 oz.)	140	36.0	0	0	0	5
Nectarine (2½″ fruit)	88	23.6	0	0	0	8

Alerts: ● Sodium ★ Sugar ■ Cholesterol

Food Description	Calories	Carbohydrates (grams)	Fat (grams)	Saturated Fat (grams)	Cholesterol (milligrams)	Sodium (milligrams)
Muskmelon balls, frozen, in syrup (12 oz.)	211	53.4	0.3	0	0	30
Orange, California Valencia (1 medium)	62	15.0	0.4	0	0	1
Orange, California Navel (1 medium)	71	17.8	0.1	0	0	1
Orange, Florida (1 medium)	71	18.1	0.3	0	0	1
Orange, mandarin, canned in water, *Nutradiet* (½ cup)	28	7.0	0	0	0	NA
★Orange, mandarin, canned, sections, *Del Monte* (5½ oz.)	100	25.0	0	0	0	10
Orange, mandarin, canned, water pack, segments, *Featherweight* (½ cup)	35	8.0	0	0	0	10
Orange, sections (1 cup)	88	22.0	0.4	0	0	2
Papaw (1)	83	16.4	0.9	0	0	3
Papaw, mashed (1 cup)	213	42.0	2.2	0	0	7
Papaya (1 medium)	119	30.4	0.3	0	0	9
Papaya, cubed (1 cup)	55	14.0	0.1	0	0	4
Peaches						
Peaches (1 lb.)	150	38.3	0.4	0	0	4
★Canned, extra light syrup, slices or halves, *Del Monte Lite* (1 cup)	100	25.0	0	0	0	NA
★Canned, grape juice pack, sliced, *Diet Delight* (½ cup)	50	14.0	0	0	0	12
★Canned, halves, *Stokely-Van Camp* (1 cup)	200	49.0	0	0	0	45
★Canned, heavy syrup, halves/slices/chunks (1 cup)	200	51.5	0.3	0	0	5
Canned, juice pack, sliced, *Libby Lite* (½ cup)	50	13.0	0	0	0	10
★Canned, slices, *Stokely-Van Camp* (1 cup)	190	48.0	0	0	0	40
Canned, water pack, halves/slices, with liquid (1 cup)	76	19.8	0.2	0	0	5
Canned, water pack, sliced, *Diet Delight* (½ cup)	30	7.0	0	0	0	12
Cling, canned in juice, halves, *Featherweight* (½ cup)	50	12.0	0	0	0	10
Cling, canned in juice, *Nutradiet* (½ cup)	60	14.0	0	0	0	NA

Alerts: ● Sodium ★ Sugar ■ Cholesterol

Food Description	Calories	Carbohydrates (grams)	Fat (grams)	Saturated Fat (grams)	Cholesterol (milligrams)	Sodium (milligrams)
Cling, canned in water, halves or slices, *Featherweight* (½ cup)	30	8.0	0	0	0	10
Cling, canned in water, *Nutradiet* (½ cup)	30	8.0	0	0	0	NA
★Dehydrated, pieces (1 cup)	340	88.0	0.9	0	0	21
★Dehydrated, pieces, prepared with sugar (1 cup)	351	90.8	0.6	0	0	14
Dried, *Del Monte* (2 oz.)	140	35.0	0	0	0	10
Freestone, canned in juice, halves or slices, *Featherweight* (½ cup)	50	12.0	0	0	0	10
Freestone, canned in juice, *Nutradiet* (½ cup)	50	14.0	0	0	0	NA
★Freestone, canned, slices or halves, *Del Monte* (1 cup)	170	45.0	0	0	0	20
★Frozen, Quick Thaw Pouch, *Birds Eye* (5 oz.)	130	34.0	0	0	0	10
★Frozen, sweetened (1 cup)	220	56.5	0.3	0	0	5
Pared (1 large fruit)	58	14.8	0.2	0	0	1
Pared, sliced (1 cup)	65	16.5	0.2	0	0	2
★Spiced, canned, *Del Monte* (7¼ oz.)	150	40.0	0	0	0	10
★Yellow cling, canned, diced, *Del Monte* (5 oz.)	110	28.0	0	0	0	10
Pears						
Pear (1 medium)	100	25.1	0.7	0	0	3
★Bartlett, canned, halves, *Libby* (1 cup)	170	44.0	0	0	0	NA
Bartlett, canned in water, halves, *Featherweight* (½ cup)	40	10.0	0	0	0	10
★Canned, extra light syrup, sliced, *Del Monte Lite* (1 cup)	110	28.0	0	0	0	NA
Canned, grape juice pack, halves or quarters, *Diet Delight* (½ cup)	60	16.0	0	0	0	12
★Canned, halves, *Stokely-Van Camp* (1 cup)	200	50.0	1.0	NA	0	30
★Canned, heavy syrup, halves or slices, *Del Monte* (1 cup)	160	43.0	0	0	0	15
★Canned, heavy syrup, halves, *S & W* (1 cup)	240	64.0	0	0	0	NA
Canned in juice, *Nutradiet* (½ cup)	60	15.0	0	0	0	NA

Alerts: •Sodium ★Sugar ■Cholesterol

Food Description	Calories	Carbohydrates (grams)	Fat (grams)	Saturated Fat (grams)	Cholesterol (milligrams)	Sodium (milligrams)
★Canned in light syrup, *Libby* (1 cup)	150	39.0	0	0	0	10
Canned in water, *Nutradiet* (½ cup)	35	10.0	0	0	0	NA
Canned, juice pack, halves, *Featherweight* (½ cup)	60	15.0	0	0	0	10
Canned, juice pack, halves, *Libby Lite* (½ cup)	60	15.0	0	0	0	10
★Canned, slices, *Stokely-Van Camp* (1 cup)	190	47.0	1.0	NA	0	20
Canned, water pack, halves, *Diet Delight* (½ cup)	35	9.0	0	0	0	12
Dried, *Del Monte* (2 oz.)	150	40.0	0	0	0	10
Dried, halves (1 cup)	482	121.1	3.2	0	0	12
Sliced or cubed (1 cup)	101	25.2	0.7	0	0	3
Persimmon, Japanese or kaki (1 large)	129	33.1	0.7	0	0	10
Persimmon, native (1 small)	31	8.2	0.1	0	0	Tr.
Pineapple						
Pineapple (1 lb.)	236	62.1	0.9	0	0	4
★Canned, chunks or crushed, in heavy syrup, *Dole* (1 cup)	189	49.5	0.3	NA	NA	3
Canned, chunks or crushed, in juice, *Dole* (1 cup)	140	35.0	1.0	NA	NA	3
★Canned, extra heavy syrup, chunk or crushed (1 cup)	234	60.8	0.3	0	0	3
Canned in juice, chunks, crushed or medium slices, *Del Monte* (1 cup)	140	35.0	0	0	0	10
Canned in juice, chunks or slices, *Featherweight* (½ cup)	70	18.0	0	0	0	10
★Canned in syrup, chunks, crushed or medium slices, *Del Monte* (1 cup)	190	49.0	0	0	0	10
Canned in water, slices, *Featherweight* (½ cup)	60	15.0	0	0	0	10
Canned in water, slices, *Nutradiet* (2 slices)	60	15.0	0	0	0	NA
Canned, water pack, tidbits, with liquid (1 cup)	96	25.1	0.2	0	0	2
Canned with juice, *Dole* (4 slices)	140	35.0	1.0	NA	NA	3
Diced (1 cup)	81	21.2	0.3	0	0	2
★Filling, *Solo* (1 oz.)	51	12.8	Tr.	0	0	7

Alerts: ● Sodium ★ Sugar ■ Cholesterol

Food Description	Calories	Carbohydrates (grams)	Fat (grams)	Saturated Fat (grams)	Cholesterol (milligrams)	Sodium (milligrams)
★Frozen, chunks, sweetened (1 cup)	208	54.4	0.2	0	0	5
Pitanga (2 fruits)	6	1.5	0	0	0	Tr.
Pitanga, pitted (1 cup)	87	21.3	0.7	0	0	3
Plantain (1 large)	313	82.0	1.1	0	0	13
Plantain (1 lb.)	540	141.5	1.8	0	0	22
Plums						
★Canned, *Del Monte* (1 cup)	190	52.0	0	0	0	10
★Canned, heavy syrup (1 cup)	214	55.8	0.3	0	0	3
★Canned in heavy syrup, *Libby* (1 cup)	210	56.0	0	0	0	10
Canned in juice, *Nutradiet* (½ cup)	80	20.0	0	0	0	NA
Canned in water, *Featherweight* (½ cup)	40	9.0	0	0	0	10
Canned, juice pack, *Featherweight* (½ cup)	80	18.0	0	0	0	10
★Canned, *Stokely-Van Camp* (1 cup)	240	60.0	0	0	0	50
Canned, water pack, whole, with liquid (1 cup)	114	29.6	0.5	0	0	5
Damson (10)	66	17.8	0	0	0	2
Damson (1 lb.)	272	73.5	0	0	0	8
Damson, halves (1 cup)	112	30.3	0	0	0	3
Prune (1)	21	5.6	0.1	0	0	Tr.
Prune (1 lb.)	320	84.0	0.9	0	0	4
Prune, halves (1 cup)	124	32.5	0.3	0	0	2
Pomegrante (1)	97	25.3	0.5	0	0	4
★Prune filling, *Solo* (1 oz.)	49	12.0	0.1	0	0	11
Prunes						
★Canned, heavy syrup, *Sunsweet* (½ cup)	120	30.0	1.0	NA	0	NA
★Canned, stewed, *Del Monte* (1 cup)	230	60.0	1.0	0	0	10
Canned, water pack, *Featherweight* (½ cup)	130	35.0	1.0	0	0	10
Dried (10 large)	215	56.9	0.5	0	0	7
Dried (10 medium)	164	43.5	0.4	0	0	5
Dried (1 lb.)	995	262.9	2.3	0	0	31
Dried, cooked without sugar, cold (1 cup)	253	66.7	0.6	0	0	8
★Dried, cooked with sugar, cold (1 cup)	409	107.3	0.5	0	0	7
Dried, *Moist-Pak, Del Monte* (2 oz.)	120	30.0	0	0	0	10

Alerts: ● Sodium ★ Sugar ■ Cholesterol

Food Description	Calories	Carbohydrates (grams)	Fat (grams)	Saturated Fat (grams)	Cholesterol (milligrams)	Sodium (milligrams)
Dried, pitted, *Del Monte* (2 oz.)	140	36.0	0	0	0	10
Dried, pitted, *Sunsweet* (2 oz.)	150	37.0	0	0	0	NA
Raisins (1 Tbsp.)	26	7.0	0	0	0	2
Raisins, chopped (1 cup)	390	104.5	0.3	0	0	36
★Raisins, cooked with sugar (1 cup)	628	166.4	0.3	0	0	38
Raisins, golden, seedless, *Del Monte* (3 oz.)	260	68.0	0	0	0	10
Raisins, ground (1 cup)	578	154.8	0.4	0	0	54
Raisins, muscat, *Del Monte* (3 oz.)	250	66.0	0	0	0	25
Raisins, Thompson seedless, *Del Monte* (3 oz.)	260	66.0	0	0	0	10
Raspberries						
Black (8 oz.)	162	35.6	3.2	0	0	2
Black (1 cup)	98	21.0	1.9	0	0	1
★Frozen in syrup, *Stokely-Van Camp* (5 oz.)	150	37.0	0	0	0	10
Red (8 oz.)	130	30.9	1.2	0	0	2
Red (1 cup)	70	16.7	0.6	0	0	1
Red, canned, water pack, with liquid (1 cup)	85	21.4	0.2	0	0	2
★Red, frozen, Quick Thaw Pouch, *Birds Eye* (5 oz.)	150	37.0	0	0	0	1
★Red, frozen, sweetened (1 cup)	245	61.5	0.5	0	0	2
★Raspberry filling, *Solo* (1 oz.)	53	13.3	Tr.	0	0	7
Rhubarb, diced (1 cup)	20	4.5	0.1	0	0	2
★Rhubarb, frozen, sweetened (10 oz.)	213	52.5	0.6	0	0	11
★Rhubarb, prepared with sugar (1 cup)	381	97.2	0.3	0	0	5
Rhubarb, well trimmed (1 lb.)	62	14.4	0.4	0	0	8
Strawberries (1 cup)	55	12.5	0.7	0	0	1
Strawberries, canned, water pack, with liquid (1 cup)	53	13.6	0.2	0	0	2
★Strawberries, frozen, halves, Quick Thaw Pouch, *Birds Eye* (5.3 oz.)	170	48.0	0	0	0	3
★Strawberries, frozen in syrup, halves, *Stokely-Van Camp* (5 oz.)	160	40.0	0	0	0	10
★Strawberries, frozen, sweetened, sliced (1 cup)	278	70.9	0.5	0	0	3

Alerts: ● Sodium ★ Sugar ■ Cholesterol

Food Description	Calories	Carbohydrates (grams)	Fat (grams)	Saturated Fat (grams)	Cholesterol (milligrams)	Sodium (milligrams)
★Strawberries, frozen, sweetened, whole (1 cup)	235	59.9	0.5	0	0	3
★Strawberries, frozen, whole, Quick Thaw Pouch, *Birds Eye* (5 oz.)	120	3.0	0	0	0	6
★Strawberry filling, *Solo* (1 oz.)	83	20.8	0	0	0	7
Tangelo (1 medium)	39	9.2	0.1	0	0	1
Tangerine (1 medium)	39	10.0	0.2	0	0	2
Tangerine, sections (1 cup)	90	22.6	0.4	0	0	4
Watermelon (1 lb.)	118	29.0	0.9	0	0	4
Watermelon, diced (1 cup)	42	10.2	0.3	0	0	2

Gelatins and Puddings

GELATINS

Food Description	Calories	Carbohydrates (grams)	Fat (grams)	Saturated Fat (grams)	Cholesterol (milligrams)	Sodium (milligrams)
●★All flavors, prepared, *Royal* (½ cup)	80	19.0	0	0	0	90
●★Apricot, prepared, *Jell-O* (½ cup)	80	19.0	0	0	0	55
●★Blackberry, prepared, *Jell-O* (½ cup)	80	19.0	0	0	0	55
●★Black raspberry, prepared, *Jell-O* (½ cup)	80	19.0	0	0	0	40
Cherry, prepared, *Carmel Kosher* (4 oz.)	8	0	0	0	0	10
●★Concord grape, prepared, *Jell-O* (½ cup)	80	19.0	0	0	0	40
Lemon, prepared, *D-Zerta* (½ cup)	8	0	0	0	0	10
●★Lemon, prepared, *Jell-O* (½ cup)	80	19.0	0	0	0	80
Lime, prepared, *D-Zerta* (½ cup)	8	0	0	0	0	7
●★Lime, prepared, *Jell-O* (½ cup)	80	18.0	0	0	0	60
●★Mixed fruit, prepared, *Jell-O* (½ cup)	80	19.0	0	0	0	55

Alerts: ● Sodium ★ Sugar ■ Cholesterol

Food Description	Calories	Carbohydrates (grams)	Fat (grams)	Saturated Fat (grams)	Cholesterol (milligrams)	Sodium (milligrams)
Orange, prepared, *Carmel Kosher* (4 oz.)	8	0	0	0	0	10
Orange, prepared, *Featherweight* (½ cup)	10	0	0	0	0	2
●★Peach, prepared, *Jell-O* (½ cup)	80	19.0	0	0	0	55
Raspberry, prepared, *Carmel Kosher* (4 oz.)	8	0	0	0	0	10
Raspberry, prepared, *Featherweight* (½ cup)	10	0	0	0	0	2
Strawberry, prepared, *D-Zerta* (½ cup)	8	0	0	0	0	8
Strawberry, prepared, *Featherweight* (½ cup)	10	0	0	0	0	2
Unflavored, *Carmel Kosher* (1 envelope)	30	0	0	0	0	0
Unflavored, dry (1 capsule)	2	0	0	0	0	Tr.
Unflavored, *Knox* (1 envelope)	25	0	0	0	0	0
●★Wild cherry, prepared, *Jell-O* (½ cup)	80	19.0	0	0	0	60
●★Wild raspberry, prepared, *Jell-O* (½ cup)	80	19.0	0	0	0	80
●★Wild strawberry, prepared, *Jell-O* (½ cup)	80	19.0	0	0	0	80
PUDDINGS						
●★Banana, canned, *Del Monte* (5 oz.)	180	30.0	5.0	NA	NA	280
●★Banana, canned, *Snack Pak* (5 oz.)	180	24.0	9.0	NA	NA	NA
●★Banana cream, *Jell-O* (¼ package)	60	14.0	0	0	0	125
●★Banana, *Royal* (¼ package)	80	20.0	1.0	0	0	140
●★Butterscotch, canned, *Del Monte* (5 oz.)	180	31.0	5.0	NA	NA	300
●Butterscotch, *D-Zerta* (⅛ package)	25	6.0	0	0	NA	85
Butterscotch, *Featherweight* (⅛ package)	12	3.0	0	0	0	5
●★Butterscotch, instant, *Jell-O* (¼ package)	100	25.0	0	0	NA	385
●★Butterscotch, *Jell-O* (¼ package)	100	24.0	0	0	0	185
Chocolate						
●★Canned, *General Mills* (½ cup)	180	30.0	5.0	NA	NA	260
D-Zerta (⅛ package)	25	6.0	0	0	0	15

Alerts: ● Sodium ★ Sugar ■ Cholesterol

Food Description	Calories	Carbohydrates (grams)	Fat (grams)	Saturated Fat (grams)	Cholesterol (milligrams)	Sodium (milligrams)
Featherweight (⅛ package)	14	2.0	0	0	0	7
●★Fudge, canned, *Del Monte* (5 oz.)	190	31.0	6.0	NA	NA	300
●★Fudge, *Jell-O* (¼ package)	100	23.0	1.0	NA	NA	130
●★German, canned, *Snack Pak,* (5 oz.)	170	25.0	7.0	NA	NA	NA
●★■Homemade (1 cup)	385	66.8	12.2	6.7	29	145
●★Instant, *Jell-O* (¼ package)	110	28.0	1.0	NA	NA	420
●★Instant, *Royal* (¼ package)	120	27.0	1.0	NA	0	NA
●★Marshmallow, canned, *Snack Pak* (5 oz.)	170	25.0	7.0	NA	NA	NA
●★Coconut, instant, *Royal* (¼ package)	100	23.0	1.0	0	0	300
●★Coffee, instant, *Royal* (¼ package)	100	24.0	1.0	0	0	225
●★■Custard, golden egg, *Americana, Jell-O* (¼ package)	90	18.0	1.0	NA	NA	120
●★■Custard, homemade (1 cup)	305	29.4	14.6	6.8	278	209
● Custard, lemon, *Sweet 'N Low* (⅛ package)	30	5.0	1.0	Tr.	5	80
●★Custard, *Royal* (¼ package)	60	15.0	0	0	0	70
● Custard, vanilla, *Sweet 'N Low* (⅛ package)	30	5.0	1.0	Tr.	5	80
●★French vanilla, instant, *Jell-O* (¼ package)	100	25.0	0	0	NA	340
●★Key lime, *Royal* (⅙ package)	50	13.0	0	0	0	100
●★Lemon, canned, *Snack Pak* (5 oz.)	150	32.0	3.0	NA	NA	NA
●★Lemon, instant, *Royal* (¼ package)	100	24.0	1.0	0	0	225
●★Pineapple cream, instant, *Jell-O* (¼ package)	100	25.0	0	0	NA	295
●★Pistachio nut, instant, *Royal* (¼ package)	100	23.0	1.0	0	0	300
●★Rice, *Americana, Jell-O* (¼ package)	100	24.0	0	0	0	100
●★Rice, canned, *General Mills* (½ cup)	150	25.0	4.0	NA	NA	150
●★Tapioca, canned, *General Mills* (½ cup)	150	22.0	5.0	NA	NA	170
●★Tapioca, chocolate, *Americana, Jell-O* (¼ package)	90	22.0	0	0	0	105

Alerts: ● Sodium ★ Sugar ■ Cholesterol

Food Description	Calories	Carbohydrates (grams)	Fat (grams)	Saturated Fat (grams)	Cholesterol (milligrams)	Sodium (milligrams)
●★Tapioca, vanilla, *Royal* (¼ package)	80	20.0	1.0	0	0	140
● Vanilla, *D-Zerta* (⅛ package)	30	7.0	0	0	NA	70
Vanilla, *Featherweight* (⅛ package)	12	3.0	0	0	0	2
●★■ Vanilla, homemade (1 cup)	283	40.5	9.9	5.5	36	165
●★ Vanilla, instant, *Jell-O* (¼ package)	80	21.0	0	0	NA	140

Gravies and Other Sauces

GRAVIES

	Calories	Carbohydrates (grams)	Fat (grams)	Saturated Fat (grams)	Cholesterol (milligrams)	Sodium (milligrams)
● Au jus, canned (10 oz.)	48	7.5	0.6	0.3	1	NA
● Au jus, canned, *Franco-American* (2 oz.)	10	2.0	0	0	0	320
● Au jus, mix, *French's* (mix for ¼ cup)	8	2.0	0	0	NA	280
●■ Bacon, with mushroom broth, canned, *Dawn Fresh* (3½ oz.)	31	5.6	0.7	Tr.	NA	522
● Beef, canned (10 oz.)	155	14.0	6.9	3.4	9	146
●■ Beef, canned, *Franco-American* (2 oz.)	30	3.0	1.0	NA	NA	290
● Brown, dehydrated (⅞ oz.)	85	14.8	2.0	1.0	2	1214
● Brown, *La Choy* (1 tsp.)	19	4.6	0.1	Tr.	Tr.	51
● Brown, mix, lite, prepared, *McCormick* (¼ cup)	10	2.0	0	0	NA	NA
● Brown, mix, *Pillsbury* (mix for ¼ cup)	15	3.0	0	0	NA	305
● Brown, mix, prepared, *Weight Watchers* (¼ cup)	8	1.0	0	0	NA	NA
● Brown, mushroom, mix, prepared, *Weight Watchers* (¼ cup)	12	2.0	0	0	NA	NA
● Brown, with onions, canned, *Franco-American* (2 oz.)	25	4.0	1.0	NA	NA	290
● Chicken, canned (10 oz.)	236	16.2	17.0	4.2	6	1718
● Chicken, canned, *Franco-American* (2 oz.)	50	3.0	4.0	NA	NA	285

Alerts: ● Sodium ★ Sugar ■ Cholesterol

Food Description	Calories	Carbohydrates (grams)	Fat (grams)	Saturated Fat (grams)	Cholesterol (milligrams)	Sodium (milligrams)
• Chicken, dehydrated (⅘ oz.)	83	14.3	1.9	0.5	2	1133
• Chicken, mix, lite, prepared, *McCormick* (¼ cup)	10	1.0	0	0	NA	NA
• Chicken, mix, *Pillsbury* (mix for ¼ cup)	15	3.0	1.0	NA	NA	220
• Home style, mix, *Pillsbury* (mix for ¼ cup)	15	3.0	0	0	NA	300
• Mushroom, canned (10 oz.)	150	16.3	8.1	1.2	0	1699
• Mushroom, canned, *Franco-American* (2 oz.)	35	4.0	2.0	NA	0	295
• Mushroom, dehydrated (¾ oz.)	70	13.8	0.9	0.5	1	1402
• Mushroom, mix, *French's* (mix for ¼ cup)	20	3.0	1.0	NA	NA	350
• Onion, dehydrated (⅚ oz.)	77	16.2	0.7	0.5	Tr.	1005
• Pork, dehydrated (¾ oz.)	76	13.4	1.9	0.8	2	1235
• Pork, mix, *French's* (mix for ¼ cup)	20	3.0	1.0	NA	NA	310
• Turkey, canned (10 oz.)	152	15.2	6.3	1.9	6	NA
• Turkey, canned, *Franco-American* (2 oz.)	30	3.0	2.0	NA	NA	330
• Turkey, dehydrated (⅞ oz.)	85	14.4	2.0	0.7	1	1421
• Turkey, mix, *French's* (mix for ¼ cup)	25	4.0	1.0	NA	NA	360
SAUCES						
• Bearnaise, mix (⅞ oz.)	90	14.8	2.2	0.3	Tr.	841
•■ Cheese, mix (1¼ oz.)	158	11.9	9.0	4.2	18	1447
•■ Cheese, mix, dry, *Tuna Helper* (⅕ package)	170	28.0	4.0	NA	NA	585
Chili, canned, *Featherweight* (1 Tbsp.)	8	2.0	0	0	0	10
• Curry, mix (1¼ oz.)	151	17.9	8.2	1.2	Tr.	1444
•■ Hollandaise, mix (1⅕ oz.)	187	10.8	15.5	9.1	40	1230
•★ Italian, canned, *Contadina* (4 oz.)	80	13.0	2.0	NA	0	556
• Marinara spaghetti, canned, *Prince* (4 oz.)	77	12.3	2.6	NA	0	587
•★ Meat flavor, canned, *Prima Salsa* (4 oz.)	120	20.0	3.0	NA	NA	NA
•★ Mushroom flavor, canned, *Prima Salsa* (4 oz.)	110	20.0	3.0	NA	0	NA
• Mushroom, mix (1 oz.)	99	15.5	2.7	0.4	0	1766
• Mushroom steak, canned, *Dawn Fresh* (3½ oz.)	31	6.2	0.3	Tr.	NA	528

Alerts: • Sodium ★ Sugar ■ Cholesterol

Food Description	Calories	Carbohydrates (grams)	Fat (grams)	Saturated Fat (grams)	Cholesterol (milligrams)	Sodium (milligrams)
●★ Pizza, canned, *Contadina* (8 oz.)	130	20.0	4.0	NA	NA	1350
●★ Spaghetti, bottled, *Prima Salsa* (1 cup)	110	20.0	3.0	NA	0	NA
Spaghetti, canned, *Featherweight* (⅔ cup)	30	10.0	3.0	NA	0	10
● Spaghetti, meatless, canned, *Prince* (4 oz.)	80	9.9	3.0	NA	0	635
●★ Spaghetti, mix (1½ oz.)	118	27.0	0.4	0.3	0	3562
●★ Spaghetti, mix, dry, *Hamburger Helper* (⅕ package)	150	31.0	1.0	NA	0	955
● Spaghetti, with meat, canned, *Prince* (4 oz.)	82	9.5	3.6	NA	NA	510
● Spaghetti, with mushrooms, canned, *Prince* (4 oz.)	77	11.2	2.6	NA	0	578
●★ Swiss steak, canned, *Contadina* (4 oz.)	40	9.0	0	0	NA	638
●★ Tomato, herb special, *Hunt-Wesson* (4 oz.)	80	12.0	4.0	NA	0	NA
●★ Tomato, special, *Hunt-Wesson* (4 oz.)	40	10.0	0	0	0	NA
●★ Tomato, with cheese, *Hunt-Wesson* (4 oz.)	70	10.0	2.0	NA	NA	NA
●★ Tomato, with mushrooms, *Del Monte* (1 cup)	100	22.0	1.0	NA	0	940
●★ Tomato, with onion, *Del Monte* (1 cup)	100	23.0	1.0	NA	0	1265
●★ Tomato, with tidbits, *Del Monte* (1 cup)	80	19.0	1.0	NA	0	1110
●★ *V-8,* canned, *Campbell's* (1 oz.)	25	6.0	1.0	NA	0	270
●■ White, medium (1 cup)	405	22.0	31.3	17.2	103	947

Ice Cream

FROZEN DESSERTS						
●★■ Assorted flavors, *Whammy, Good Humor* (1.6 oz.)	100	9.0	7.0	NA	NA	NA

Alerts: ● Sodium ★ Sugar ■ Cholesterol

Food Description	Calories	Carbohydrates (grams)	Fat (grams)	Saturated Fat (grams)	Cholesterol (milligrams)	Sodium (milligrams)
●★■ Chip crunch, *Whammy, Good Humor* (1.6 oz.)	110	10.0	7.0	NA	NA	NA
●★■ Chocolate coated, vanilla, *Good Humor* (3 oz.)	170	12.0	13.0	NA	NA	NA
●★■ Chocolate eclair, *Good Humor* (3 oz.)	220	25.0	13.0	NA	NA	NA
●★■ Ice cream sandwich, *Good Humor* (2.5 oz.)	200	34.0	6.0	NA	NA	NA
★ Ice, lime (1 cup)	247	62.9	0	0	0	0
●★■ Ice, *Whammy, Good Humor* (1.5 oz.)	50	13.0	0	0	0	NA
★ Sherbet, orange (1 cup)	259	59.4	2.3	0	0	19
●★■ Strawberry shortcake, *Good Humor* (3 oz.)	200	21.0	13.0	NA	NA	NA
●★■ Toasted almond, *Good Humor* (3 oz.)	220	21.0	14.0	NA	NA	NA
ICE CREAM						
●★■ Black cherry, *Good Humor* (4 oz.)	130	14.0	8.0	NA	NA	NA
●★ Butter almond, *Breyers* (4 oz.)	170	15.0	10.0	4.4	23	42
●★■ Butter pecan, *Good Humor* (4 oz.)	150	14.0	9.0	NA	NA	NA
●★ Cherry vanilla, *Breyers* (½ cup)	140	17.0	7.0	3.8	20	40
●★■ Chocolate chip, *Good Humor* (4 oz.)	150	15.0	8.0	NA	NA	NA
●★■ Chocolate, *Good Humor* (4 oz.)	130	15.0	7.0	NA	NA	NA
●★■ Fudge, royal, *Good Humor* (4 oz.)	120	14.0	6.0	NA	NA	NA
●★ Natural vanilla with bean specks, *Breyers* (½ cup)	150	15.0	8.0	4.3	23	45
●★ Neapolitan, *Breyers* (½ cup)	150	17.0	8.0	4.0	20	36
●★■ Neapolitan, *Good Humor* (4 oz.)	130	14.0	7.0	NA	NA	NA
★ 16% fat (1 cup)	329	26.6	23.8	13.1	84	48
●★■ Strawberry, *Good Humor* (4 oz.)	120	15.0	6.0	NA	NA	NA
●★■ 10% fat (1 cup)	257	27.7	14.1	7.8	53	83
●★■ 10% fat, soft serve (1 cup)	334	36.0	18.3	10.1	69	109
●★■ Toffee fudge swirl, *Good Humor* (4 oz.)	130	18.0	7.0	NA	NA	NA
●★■ Vanilla fudge swirl, *Good Humor* (4 oz.)	140	15.0	8.0	NA	NA	NA
●★■ Vanilla, *Good Humor* (4 oz.)	140	14.0	8.0	NA	NA	NA

Alerts: ● Sodium ★ Sugar ■ Cholesterol

Food Description	Calories	Carbohydrates (grams)	Fat (grams)	Saturated Fat (grams)	Cholesterol (milligrams)	Sodium (milligrams)
ICE MILK						
●★Butter almond, *Sweet 'N Low* (4 oz.)	120	13.0	6.0	NA	NA	NA
●★Butter pecan, *Sweet 'N Low* (4 oz.)	120	13.0	6.0	NA	NA	NA
●★Chocolate, *Sweet 'N Low* (4 oz.)	100	14.0	3.0	NA	NA	NA
●★5.1% fat (1 cup)	199	29.3	6.7	3.7	26	89
●★5.1% fat, soft serve (1 cup)	266	39.2	8.9	4.9	35	119
●★Imitation, chocolate, *Weight Watchers* (3 oz.)	100	19.0	1.0	NA	2	70
●★Imitation, coffee, *Weight Watchers* (3 oz.)	100	19.0	1.0	NA	2	70
●★Imitation, lemon, *Weight Watchers* (3 oz.)	100	19.0	1.0	NA	2	70
●★Imitation, maple, *Weight Watchers* (3 oz.)	100	19.0	1.0	NA	2	70
●★Imitation, mint, *Weight Watchers* (3 oz.)	100	19.0	1.0	NA	2	70
●★Imitation, neapolitan, *Weight Watchers* (3 oz.)	100	19.0	1.0	NA	2	70
●★Imitation, strawberry, *Weight Watchers* (3 oz.)	100	19.0	1.0	NA	2	70
●★Imitation, vanilla, *Weight Watchers* (3 oz.)	100	19.0	1.0	NA	2	70
●★Lemon chiffon, *Sweet 'N Low* (4 oz.)	100	14.0	3.0	NA	NA	NA
●★Strawberry, *Sweet 'N Low* (4 oz.)	100	14.0	3.0	NA	NA	NA
●★Vanilla fudge, *Sweet 'N Low* (4 oz.)	100	14.0	3.0	NA	NA	NA
●★Vanilla, *Sweet 'N Low* (4 oz.)	100	14.0	3.0	NA	NA	NA

Alerts: ● Sodium ★ Sugar ■ Cholesterol

Jellies and Jams

Food Description	Calories	Carbohydrates (grams)	Fat (grams)	Saturated Fat (grams)	Cholesterol (milligrams)	Sodium (milligrams)
★Apple butter (1 Tbsp.)	33	8.2	0.1	0	0	Tr.
★Apple butter, natural cider, *Smucker's* (2 tsp.)	25	6.0	0	0	0	Tr.
★Apple butter, natural, *Smucker's* (2 tsp.)	25	6.0	0	0	0	Tr.
★Jam, all flavors, calorie reduced, *Nutradiet* (1 tsp.)	4	1.0	0	0	0	NA
★Jam, all flavors, imitation, low calorie, *Slenderella* (2 tsp.)	16	4.0	0	0	0	NA
★Jam, all flavors, *Smucker's* (2 tsp.)	35	9.0	0	0	0	Tr.
★Jam, all fruit flavors (1 Tbsp.)	54	14.0	0	0	0	2
★Jam, grape, *Welch's* (2 tsp.)	35	9.0	0	0	0	Tr.
Jam, strawberry, imitation, artificially sweetened, *Smucker's* (2 tsp.)	2	2.0	0	0	0	10
★Jam, strawberry, *Welch's* (2 tsp.)	35	9.0	0	0	0	Tr.
Jellies						
★All flavors (1 Tbsp.)	49	12.7	0	0	0	3
All flavors, artificially sweetened, *Featherweight* (1 Tbsp.)	6	1.0	0	0	0	NA
★All flavors, imitation, calorie reduced, *Featherweight* (1 Tbsp.)	16	4.0	0	0	0	NA
★All flavors, imitation, low calorie, *Slenderella* (2 tsp.)	16	4.0	0	0	0	NA
★All flavors, *Smucker's* (2 tsp.)	35	9.0	0	0	0	Tr.
★Apple, imitation, low calorie, *Spred Lite* (1 tsp.)	7	2.0	0	0	0	NA
★Concord grape, calorie reduced *Nutradiet* (1 tsp.)	4	1.0	0	0	0	NA
Grape, imitation, artificially sweetened, *Smucker's* (2 tsp.)	2	2.0	0	0	0	10

Alerts: ● Sodium ★ Sugar ■ Cholesterol

Food Description	Calories	Carbohydrates (grams)	Fat (grams)	Saturated Fat (grams)	Cholesterol (milligrams)	Sodium (milligrams)
★Grape, imitation, low calorie, *Spred Lite* (1 tsp.)	7	2.0	0	0	0	NA
★Grape, *Welch's* (2 tsp.)	35	9.0	0	0	0	Tr.
★Marmalade, citrus (1 Tbsp.)	51	14.0	0	0	0	3
★Marmalade, orange, calorie reduced, *Nutradiet* (1 tsp.)	4	1.0	0	0	0	NA
★Marmalade, orange, *Featherweight* (1 Tbsp.)	16	4.0	0	0	0	NA
★Marmalade, orange, sweet, *Smucker's* (2 tsp.)	35	9.0	0	0	0	Tr.
★Peach butter, *Smucker's* (2 tsp.)	30	8.0	0	0	0	Tr.
Preserves						
All flavors, artificially sweetened, *Featherweight* (1 Tbsp.)	6	1.0	0	0	0	NA
★All flavors, calorie reduced, *Nutradiet* (1 tsp.)	4	1.0	0	0	0	NA
★All flavors, *Featherweight* (1 Tbsp.)	16	4.0	0	0	0	NA
★All flavors, *Smucker's* (2 tsp.)	35	9.0	0	0	0	Tr.
★All fruit flavors (1 Tbsp.)	54	14.0	0	0	0	2
★Grape, *Welch's* (2 tsp.)	35	9.0	0	0	0	Tr.
★Strawberry, imitation, low calorie, *Spred Lite* (1 tsp.)	5	1.0	0	0	0	NA
★Strawberry, *Welch's* (2 tsp.)	35	9.0	0	0	0	Tr.
★Spread, grape, *Lite, Welch's* (2 tsp.)	20	5.0	0	0	0	NA
★Spread, strawberry, *Lite, Welch's* (2 tsp.)	20	5.0	0	0	0	NA

Meals and Entrees

ENTREES						
●★Beans and franks, canned (1 cup)	367	32.1	18.1	7.7	33	1374
●★Canelloni, frozen, *Weight Watchers* (13 oz.)	450	54.0	12.0	NA	88	1015

Alerts: ● Sodium ★ Sugar ■ Cholesterol

Food Description	Calories	Carbohydrates (grams)	Fat (grams)	Saturated Fat (grams)	Cholesterol (milligrams)	Sodium (milligrams)
● Beef, chipped, creamed, frozen, *Banquet* (5 oz.)	124	10.5	4.1	NA	NA	949
● Beef, chipped, creamed, frozen, *Morton Boil-in-Bag* (5 oz.)	160	9.0	9.0	NA	17	1370
● Beef patties, with mushroom gravy, frozen, *Morton* (8 oz.)	300	12.0	20.0	NA	54	1170
● Beef, short ribs, boneless, with vegetable gravy, frozen, *Stouffers* (5¾ oz.)	350	2.0	25.0	NA	NA	560
● Beef, sliced, frozen, *Swanson Hungry-Man* (12¼ oz.)	330	23.0	9.0	NA	NA	850
●■ Brains, pork, with milk gravy, canned, *Armour* (2¾ oz.)	100	0	8.0	NA	NA	453
●★ Cabbage rolls, stuffed with beef, in tomato sauce, frozen, *Green Giant* (3½ oz.)	105	8.0	5.6	NA	NA	483
● Chicken a la king, canned, *Swanson* (5¼ oz.)	180	9.0	12.0	NA	NA	681
● Chicken a la king, frozen, *Banquet* (5 oz.)	138	10.4	4.7	NA	NA	892
● Chicken a la king, frozen, *Green Giant Toast Topper* (3½ oz.)	114	5.4	6.5	NA	NA	600
● Chicken and dumplings, canned, *Swanson* (7½ oz.)	220	18.0	12.0	NA	NA	1030
● Chicken, with wine sauce, frozen, *Swanson* (8¼ oz.)	370	10.0	27.0	NA	NA	1060
●★ Chili con carne, with beans, canned, *Swanson* (7¾ oz.)	310	28.0	15.0	NA	NA	1100
●★ Chili con carne, with beans, frozen *Weight Watchers* (10 oz.)	330	34.0	12.0	NA	NA	769
●★ Chili, Mexican-style, *Stokely-Van Camp* (1 cup)	240	44.0	3.0	NA	NA	820
●★ Chili, with beans, canned, *Armour* (7¾ oz.)	360	28.0	21.0	NA	NA	911
★ Chili, with beans, canned, *Featherweight* (7½ oz.)	270	25.0	12.0	NA	NA	75
●★ Chili, with beans, canned, *Stokely-Van Camp* (1 cup)	390	24.0	26.0	NA	NA	1260
●★ Chili, w/o beans, canned, *Armour* (7½ oz.)	390	12.0	31.0	NA	NA	921
●★ Chop suey, beef, frozen, *Banquet* (7 oz.)	73	9.5	1.4	NA	NA	1140

Alerts: ● Sodium ★ Sugar ■ Cholesterol

Food Description	Calories	Carbohydrates (grams)	Fat (grams)	Saturated Fat (grams)	Cholesterol (milligrams)	Sodium (milligrams)
• Chop suey, with meat, no noodles, homemade (1 cup)	300	12.8	17.0	8.5	100	1052
•★ Chow mein, chicken, frozen, *La Choy* (1 cup)	68	5.0	2.3	NA	14	924
•★ Chow mein, meatless, frozen, *La Choy* (1 cup)	47	5.9	1.4	NA	1	835
•★ Chow mein, pepper oriental, frozen, *La Choy* (1 cup)	89	10.2	1.4	NA	16	1024
•★ Chow mein, shrimp, frozen, *La Choy* (1 cup)	61	5.7	1.6	NA	40	951
•★ Crepes, chicken, with mushroom sauce, frozen, *Stouffers* (8¼ oz.)	390	19.0	22.0	NA	NA	1040
•★ Crepes, crab, frozen, *Mrs. Paul* (5½ oz.)	240	24.0	12.0	NA	NA	1155
•★ Crepes, mushroom, frozen, *Stouffers* (6¼ oz.)	255	27.0	13.0	NA	NA	865
•★ Crepes, shrimp, frozen, *Mrs. Paul* (5½ oz.)	250	24.0	12.0	NA	NA	1045
Dumplings, stuffed with chicken, canned, *Featherweight* (7½ oz.)	160	18.0	4.0	NA	NA	85
•★ Eggplant parmigiana, frozen, *Weight Watchers* (13 oz.)	280	25.0	13.0	NA	57	473
•★ Enchilada, beef, frozen, *Swanson* (11¼ oz.)	450	42.0	24.0	NA	NA	NA
• Fish, au gratin, frozen, *Mrs. Paul* (5 oz.)	250	23.0	12.0	NA	NA	850
• Gravy and sliced beef, frozen, *Banquet* (5 oz.)	116	4.8	4.3	NA	NA	852
• Green pepper, stuffed with beef and crumbs (6½ oz.)	314	31.1	10.2	4.8	70	580
•★ Green peppers, stuffed with beef, in creole sauce, frozen, *Green Giant* (3½ oz.)	101	9.0	5.0	NA	NA	462
• Hash, corned beef, canned (1 cup)	398	23.5	24.9	11.9	73	1188
• Hash, corned beef, canned, *Armour* (7½ oz.)	400	19.0	28.0	NA	NA	1212
• Lasagna, frozen, *Stouffers* (10½ oz.)	385	36.0	14.0	NA	NA	1200
•■ Lasagna, frozen, *Weight Watchers* (13 oz.)	350	39.0	10.0	NA	152	665
•★ Meat loaf, with tomato sauce, frozen, *Morton* (8 oz.)	200	17.0	8.0	NA	53	1100

Alerts: • Sodium ★ Sugar ■ Cholesterol

Food Description	Calories	Carbohydrates (grams)	Fat (grams)	Saturated Fat (grams)	Cholesterol (milligrams)	Sodium (milligrams)
●■Pepper, veal-stuffed, frozen, *Weight Watchers* (13 oz.)	320	29.0	9.0	NA	144	960
●★Pierogies, cabbage, frozen, *Mrs. Paul* (5 oz.)	330	63.0	4.0	NA	NA	650
●★Pierogies, potato and cheese, frozen, *Mrs. Paul* (5 oz.)	300	56.0	4.0	NA	NA	550
●★Pierogies, sauerkraut, Polish style, frozen, *Mrs. Paul* (5 oz.)	310	60.0	3.0	NA	NA	400
Potpies						
●★Beef, frozen, *Swanson Hungry-Man* (16 oz.)	770	65.0	44.0	NA	NA	2155
●★Beef, homemade (7.4 oz.)	517	39.5	30.4	8.4	44	596
●★Chicken, frozen, *Morton* (8 oz.)	320	33.0	13.0	NA	36	1246
●★Chicken, homemade (8.2 oz.)	545	42.5	31.3	10.9	72	593
●★Steak burger, frozen, *Swanson Hungry-Man* (16 oz.)	830	69.0	50.0	NA	NA	1675
●★Tuna, frozen, *Morton* (8 oz.)	370	36.0	18.0	NA	33	1120
●★Turkey, frozen, *Swanson Hungry-Man* (16 oz.)	800	64.0	47.0	NA	NA	2020
●★Turkey, homemade (8.2 oz.)	550	42.9	31.3	10.5	72	633
●★Sloppy Joes, canned, *Armour* (7.6 oz.)	330	25.0	20.0	NA	NA	1433
●★Sloppy Joes, frozen, *Green Giant Toast Topper* (3½ oz.)	108	10.1	4.0	NA	NA	800
●★Sloppy Joes, pork, canned, *Armour* (7.6 oz.)	350	22.0	23.0	NA	NA	1357
●■Souffle, cheese, frozen, *Stouffers* (6 oz.)	355	14.0	26.0	NA	NA	1360
●★Steak and green peppers, in oriental style sauce, frozen, *Swanson* (8½ oz.)	200	11.0	9.0	NA	NA	855
●Steak, salisbury, with gravy, frozen, *Green Giant* (3½ oz.)	138	7.0	8.0	NA	NA	512
●Stew, beef and vegetable, canned (1 cup)	194	17.4	7.6	2.5	34	1006
●Stew, beef, canned, *Swanson* (7½ oz.)	190	18.0	7.0	NA	NA	965
●Stew, beef, frozen, *Green Giant* (3½ oz.)	65	7.9	1.1	NA	NA	375
★Stew, beef, low sodium, canned, *Featherweight* (7¼ oz.)	210	24.0	8.0	NA	NA	50

Alerts: ● Sodium ★ Sugar ■ Cholesterol

Food Description	Calories	Carbohydrates (grams)	Fat (grams)	Saturated Fat (grams)	Cholesterol (milligrams)	Sodium (milligrams)
• Stew, beef, with biscuits, frozen, *Green Giant* (3½ oz.)	92	10.2	2.6	NA	NA	432
• Stew, chicken, canned, *Swanson* (7½ oz.)	160	16.0	7.0	NA	NA	910
★ Stew, chicken, low sodium, canned, *Featherweight* (7½ oz.)	170	20.0	6.0	NA	NA	55
• Stroganoff, beef, with parsley noodles, frozen, *Stouffers* (9¾ oz.)	390	31.0	20.0	NA	NA	1300
• Tamales, beef, canned, *Armour* (6¾ oz.)	350	28.0	23.0	NA	NA	NA
•■ Tripe, beef, canned, *Armour* (6 oz.)	310	3.0	23.0	NA	NA	216
• Tuna noodle casserole, frozen, *Stouffers* (5¾ oz.)	200	18.0	9.0	NA	NA	670
• Turkey croquettes, with gravy, frozen, *Morton* (8 oz.)	440	30.0	26.0	NA	42	1360
• Turkey tetrazzini, frozen, *Stouffers* (6 oz.)	240	17.0	14.0	NA	NA	620
• Turkey tetrazzini, frozen, *Weight Watchers* (13 oz.)	380	43.0	8.0	NA	42	1225
• Turkey, with gravy, frozen, *Morton* (8 oz.)	200	8.0	10.0	NA	38	1120
•★ Veal parmigiana, frozen, *Banquet* (5 oz.)	287	19.5	16.2	NA	NA	1014
•★ Veal parmigiana, frozen, *Morton* (8 oz.)	300	25.0	14.0	NA	49	1180
•★ Veal parmigiana, frozen, *Morton Boil-in-Bag* (5 oz.)	130	14.0	4.0	NA	24	580
•■ Welsh rarebit, frozen, *Green Giant Toast Topper* (3½ oz.)	154	8.0	10.4	NA	NA	NA
•■ Welsh rarebit, frozen, *Stouffers* (5 oz.)	355	17.0	29.0	NA	NA	660
•■ Welsh rarebit, homemade (1 cup)	415	14.6	31.6	17.3	100	770
FROZEN MEALS						
•★ Beans and franks, *Swanson* (11¼ oz.)	550	75.0	19.0	NA	NA	1370
•★■ Beef, chopped, *Swanson Hungry-Man* (18 oz.)	730	70.0	41.0	NA	NA	2065
•★■ Beef, sliced, *Swanson Hungry-Man* (17 oz.)	540	51.0	18.0	NA	NA	1365
• Beefsteak, *Weight Watchers* (10 oz.)	390	17.0	24.0	NA	99	730

Alerts: • Sodium ★ Sugar ■ Cholesterol

Food Description	Calories	Carbohydrates (grams)	Fat (grams)	Saturated Fat (grams)	Cholesterol (milligrams)	Sodium (milligrams)
Chicken						
●★Banquet Man Pleaser (17 oz.)	1026	89.2	51.6	NA	NA	3562
● Boneless, Morton (10 oz.)	230	24.0	6.0	NA	48	1350
●★Boneless, Swanson Hungry-Man (19 oz.)	730	74.0	29.0	NA	NA	2180
● Fried, Banquet (11 oz.)	530	48.4	25.0	NA	NA	2371
●★Fried, barbecue flavored, Swanson (11¼ oz.)	530	47.0	29.0	NA	NA	845
●★Fried, Morton (15 oz.)	710	96.0	18.0	NA	98	2180
●■Livers and onions, Weight Watchers (10½ oz.)	220	15.0	5.0	NA	480	1030
●★Oriental, Weight Watchers (15 oz.)	320	31.0	6.0	NA	166	2260
● Parmigiana, Weight Watchers (9 oz.)	200	8.0	9.0	NA	59	830
●■Eggs, scrambled with sausage and hash browns, Swanson (6¼ oz.)	460	22.0	31.0	NA	NA	675
●★Enchiladas, beef, Morton (11 oz.)	280	44.0	6.0	NA	18	1216
●★Enchiladas, beef, Swanson (15 oz.)	570	72.0	27.0	NA	NA	1575
● Fish and chips, light batter, frozen, Mrs. Paul (7 oz.)	370	45.0	16.0	NA	NA	1050
● Fish and chips, Swanson (10¼ oz.)	450	38.0	22.0	NA	NA	695
● Flounder, with lemon flavored bread crumbs, Weight Watchers (8½ oz.)	160	13.0	2.0	NA	54	538
●★■French toast, with sausage, Swanson (4½ oz.)	300	22.0	17.0	NA	NA	665
●★German style, Swanson (11¾ oz.)	430	40.0	17.0	NA	NA	1465
● Haddock, with stuffing, Weight Watchers (8¾ oz.)	180	14.0	2.0	NA	103	657
●★Ham, Morton (10 oz.)	440	57.0	17.0	NA	64	1865
●★Meat loaf, Banquet (11 oz.)	412	29.0	23.7	NA	NA	1991
●★Meat loaf, Morton (11 oz.)	340	28.0	15.0	NA	61	1380
●★Mexican style combination, Swanson (16 oz.)	700	75.0	35.0	NA	NA	1790
●★Mexican style, Morton (11 oz.)	300	45.0	8.0	NA	16	1242
●★Pancakes and sausage, Swanson (6 oz.)	500	50.0	25.0	NA	NA	1050

Alerts: ● Sodium ★ Sugar ■ Cholesterol

Food Description	Calories	Carbohydrates (grams)	Fat (grams)	Saturated Fat (grams)	Cholesterol (milligrams)	Sodium (milligrams)
● Perch, with lemon flavored bread crumbs, *Weight Watchers* (8½ oz.)	190	9.0	5.0	NA	108	577
● ★ Polynesian style, *Swanson* (13 oz.)	490	65.0	17.0	NA	NA	1730
● ★ Pork loin, *Swanson* (11¼ oz.)	470	48.0	22.0	NA	NA	795
● Sole, with lobster sauce, *Weight Watchers* (9½ oz.)	200	17.0	3.0	NA	91	614
● ★ Steak, salisbury, *Swanson Hungry-Man* (17 oz.)	870	63.0	51.0	NA	NA	1760
● ★ Steak, salisbury, 3 courses, *Swanson* (16 oz.)	490	47.0	23.0	NA	NA	1680
● ★ Steak, Swiss, *Swanson* (10 oz.)	350	40.0	13.0	NA	NA	965
● Turkey, *Banquet* (11 oz.)	293	27.8	9.7	NA	NA	1797
● Turkey breast, sliced, *Weight Watchers* (16 oz.)	400	32.0	12.0	NA	134	1440
● ★ Turkey, *Morton* (19 oz.)	580	65.0	21.0	NA	75	2567
● Turkey, sliced, *Morton* (15 oz.)	520	80.0	13.0	NA	45	1722
● ★ Turkey, 3 courses, *Swanson* (16 oz.)	520	62.0	19.0	NA	NA	1700
● ★ Veal parmigiana, *Morton* (20 oz.)	600	83.0	15.0	NA	72	2430
● ★ Veal parmigiana, *Swanson* (12¼ oz.)	510	51.0	25.0	NA	NA	1110
● ★ Western style, *Morton* (11⁴/₅ oz.)	400	32.0	23.0	NA	52	1650
● ★ Western style, *Swanson* (11¾ oz.)	440	42.0	21.0	NA	NA	1060
PIZZAS						
● ★ ■ Cheese (⅛ of pie)	147	21.8	4.1	1.5	11	379
● ★ ■ Cheese, extra, *Totino's* (½ pizza)	560	48.0	34.0	NA	NA	1150
● ★ ■ Cheese, frozen (2 oz.)	140	20.2	4.0	1.5	10	368
● ★ ■ Cheese, frozen, *John's Original* (5⅓ oz.)	410	45.0	17.0	NA	NA	NA
● ★ ■ Cheese, frozen, *La Pizzeria* (5 oz.)	290	33.0	11.0	8.0	20	770
● ★ ■ Cheese, homemade (⅛ pie)	153	18.4	5.4	2.1	12	456
● ★ ■ Cheese, thick crust, frozen, *La Pizzeria* (6.2 oz.)	410	46.0	15.0	8.0	30	970
● ★ ■ Combination, frozen, *La Pizzeria* (6¾ oz.)	450	46.0	20.0	10.0	35	1140

Alerts: ● Sodium ★ Sugar ■ Cholesterol

Food Description	Calories	Carbohydrates (grams)	Fat (grams)	Saturated Fat (grams)	Cholesterol (milligrams)	Sodium (milligrams)
●★■ Deluxe, frozen, *Celeste* (5.9 oz.)	360	36.0	17.0	NA	NA	NA
●★■ Deluxe, frozen, *John's Original* (7 oz.)	450	54.0	16.0	NA	NA	NA
●★■ Deluxe, Sicilian style, frozen, *Celeste* (6 oz.)	425	43.8	19.5	NA	NA	NA
●★■ French bread, cheese, frozen, *Stouffers* (5.1 oz.)	330	43.0	13.0	NA	NA	850
●★■ French bread, deluxe, frozen, *Stouffers* (6.2 oz.)	400	46.0	18.0	NA	NA	1150
●★■ French bread, hamburger, frozen, *Stouffers* (6.1 oz.)	400	39.0	20.0	NA	NA	1100
●★■ French bread, sausage and mushroom, frozen, *Stouffers* (6¼ oz.)	395	40.0	18.0	NA	NA	1220
●★ Mix, regular, *Appian Way* (6¼ oz.)	370	73.0	7.0	NA	NA	810
●★ Mix, thick crust, *Appian Way* (7 oz.)	500	86.0	11.0	NA	NA	949
●★■ Pepperoni and mushroom, frozen, *Totino's* (⅓ pizza)	510	40.0	33.0	NA	NA	990
●★■ Pepperoni, frozen, *Celeste* (5 oz.)	350	32.0	17.0	NA	NA	NA
●★■ Pepperoni, frozen, *La Pizzeria* (5¼ oz.)	360	39.0	14.0	6.0	40	920
●★■ Sausage and pepperoni, Chicago style, frozen, *Celeste* (6 oz.)	400	36.0	21.0	NA	NA	NA
●★■ Sausage and pepperoni, frozen, *Totino's* (⅓ pizza)	530	39.0	35.0	NA	NA	1000
●★■ Sausage, Chicago style, frozen, *Celeste* (6 oz.)	420	38.0	22.0	NA	NA	NA
●★■ Sausage, frozen, *John's Original* (5⅓ oz.)	410	47.0	17.0	NA	NA	NA
●★■ Sausage, frozen, *La Pizzeria* (6½ oz.)	420	47.0	17.0	9.0	30	1020
●★■ Sausage, homemade (⅛ pie)	157	19.8	6.2	1.8	13	488
●★ Topping, *Appian Way* (6 oz.)	100	11.0	6.0	NA	NA	NA

Alerts: ● Sodium ★ Sugar ■ Cholesterol

Meats

All meats contain cholesterol and sodium in varying, yet *relatively* substantial, amounts. If you are restricting either of these two food constituents in your diet, you should maintain an awareness of your cholesterol or sodium intake when you consume meat. We have assigned an alert to a particular item only when the cholesterol or sodium content may be considered unacceptably high—due to the nature of the food or the method of processing or preparation—when compared to other meat items.

Food Description	Calories	Carbohydrates (grams)	Fat (grams)	Saturated Fat (grams)	Cholesterol (milligrams)	Sodium (milligrams)
Beaver, roasted (3 oz.)	211	0	11.6	4.3	85	34
Rabbit, stewed, diced (1 cup)	302	0	14.1	5.6	127	57
Rabbit, stewed (8.6 oz./yield of 1 lb. ready-to-cook)	529	0	24.7	9.8	223	100
Venison, raw (3 oz.)	107	0	3.4	2.1	55	76
BEEF						
• Breakfast strips, *Lean 'n Tasty* (1 strip)	40	0.2	3.0	1.3	11	202
Chuck roast, round-bone, braised, drained (3 oz. slice)	246	0	16.3	7.8	80	40
Chuck roast, round-bone, braised, drained, trimmed of fat (3 oz. slice)	164	0	5.9	2.9	77	45
Chuck roast, round-bone in, braised, drained (9.5 oz./yield of 1 lb. raw)	780	0	51.8	24.9	254	128
Chuck roast, round-bone in, braised, drained, trimmed of fat (8.1 oz./yield of 1 lb. raw)	444	0	16.1	7.7	209	122
Chuck steak, blade cut, bone in, braised, drained (9 oz./yield of 1 lb. raw)	1089	0	93.6	44.9	240	100
Chuck steak, blade cut, bone in, braised, drained, trimmed of fat (6.2 oz./yield of 1 lb. raw)	438	0	24.5	11.7	160	89

Alerts: • Sodium ★ Sugar ■ Cholesterol

Food Description	Calories	Carbohydrates (grams)	Fat (grams)	Saturated Fat (grams)	Cholesterol (milligrams)	Sodium (milligrams)
Chuck steak, blade cut, braised, drained (3 oz. piece)	363	0	31.2	15.0	80	33
Chuck steak, blade cut, braised, drained, trimmed of fat (3 oz. piece)	212	0	11.8	5.7	77	43
Chuck stew meat, cooked, chopped or diced (1 cup)	458	0	33.5	16.1	132	63
Chuck stew meat, cooked, drained (10.7 oz./yield of 1 lb. raw)	994	0	72.7	34.9	286	138
Chuck stew meat, cooked, drained, trimmed of fat (10.7 oz./yield of 1 lb. raw)	651	0	28.9	13.9	277	159
Club steak, bone in, broiled (9.8 oz./yield of 1 lb. raw)	1262	0	112.9	54.2	261	140
Club steak, bone in, broiled, trimmed of fat (5.7 oz./yield of 1 lb. raw)	393	0	20.9	10.1	147	116
Club steak, boneless, broiled (11.7 oz./yield of 1 lb. raw)	1503	0	134.4	64.5	311	167
Club steak, boneless, broiled, trimmed of fat (6.8 oz./yield of 1 lb. raw)	468	0	25.0	12.0	175	139
● Corned beef, cooked (10.7 oz./yield of 1 lb. uncooked)	1131	0	92.4	44.4	286	2866
● Corned beef, cooked (3 oz. slice)	316	0	25.9	12.4	80	802
Flank steak, braised, drained (10.7 oz./yield of 1 lb. raw)	596	0	22.2	10.6	286	162
Flank steak, braised, drained (3 oz. slice)	167	0	6.2	3.0	80	45
Hamburger/10% fat, broiled (12 oz./yield of 1 lb. raw)	745	0	38.4	18.4	320	228
Hamburger/10% fat, raw (1 lb.)	812	0	45.4	21.8	308	328
Hamburger/21% fat, broiled (11.5 oz./yield of 1 lb. raw)	932	0	66.2	31.8	306	193
■ Heart, braised, diced (1 cup)	273	1.0	8.3	4.4	397	150
■ Kidney, braised (4 oz.)	286	0.9	13.6	3.4	912	287
■ Liver, fried (3 oz. slice)	195	4.5	9.0	2.6	372	156
Porterhouse steak, broiled (10.6 oz./yield of 1 lb. raw)	1400	0	127.0	61.0	283	145

Alerts: ● Sodium ★ Sugar ■ Cholesterol

Food Description	Calories	Carbohydrates (grams)	Fat (grams)	Saturated Fat (grams)	Cholesterol (milligrams)	Sodium (milligrams)
Porterhouse steak, broiled (3 oz. piece)	395	0	35.9	17.2	80	41
Porterhouse steak, broiled, trimmed of fat (6.1 oz./yield of 1 lb. raw)	385	0	18.1	8.7	157	127
Rib roast, bone in, roasted (10.7 oz./yield of 1 lb. raw)	1342	0	120.2	57.7	287	148
Rib roast, bone in, roasted (3 oz. slice)	374	0	33.5	16.1	80	41
Rib roast, bone in, roasted, trimmed of fat (6.9 oz./yield of 1 lb. raw)	470	0	26.1	12.5	117	134
Rib roast, bone in, roasted, trimmed of fat (3 oz. slice)	205	0	11.4	5.5	77	58
Round steak, bone in, braised or broiled (10.7 oz./yield of 1 lb. raw)	793	0	46.8	22.5	286	213
Round steak, braised or broiled (3 oz. piece)	222	0	13.1	6.3	80	60
Round steak, bone in, braised or broiled, trimmed of fat (9.2 oz./yield of 1 lb. raw)	491	0	15.9	7.6	237	199
Round steak, braised or broiled, trimmed of fat (3 oz. piece)	161	0	5.2	2.5	77	65
Rump roast, bone in, roasted (9.9 oz./yield of 1 lb. raw)	975	0	76.7	36.8	264	162
Rump roast, bone in, roasted, trimmed of fat (7.4 oz./yield of 1 lb. raw)	439	0	19.6	9.4	192	150
Rump roast, boneless, roasted (11.7 oz./yield of 1 lb. raw)	1149	0	90.4	43.4	311	191
Rump roast, boneless, roasted, trimmed of fat (8.8 oz./yield of 1 lb. raw)	516	0	23.1	11.1	226	176
Rump roast, roasted (3 oz. slice)	295	0	23.2	11.1	80	49
Rump roast, roasted, trimmed of fat (3 oz. slice)	177	0	7.9	3.8	77	61
Short plate, bone in, simmered, drained (9.3 oz./yield of 1 lb. raw)	1140	0	98.5	47.3	248	103

Alerts: • Sodium ★ Sugar ■ Cholesterol

Food Description	Calories	Carbohydrates (grams)	Fat (grams)	Saturated Fat (grams)	Cholesterol (milligrams)	Sodium (milligrams)
Short plate, bone in, simmered, drained, trimmed of fat (5.7 oz./yield of 1 lb. raw)	320	0	12.4	6.0	147	85
Sirloin Steak						
Flat-bone, broiled (3 oz. piece)	347	0	29.5	14.2	80	46
Flat-bone, broiled, trimmed of fat (3 oz. piece)	184	0	8.1	3.9	77	64
Flat-bone in, broiled (9.6 oz./yield of 1 lb. raw)	1110	0	94.4	45.3	256	148
Flat-bone in, broiled, trimmed of fat (6.3 oz./yield of 1 lb. raw)	387	0	17.0	8.2	163	134
Pinbone, broiled (3 oz. piece)	414	0	38.2	18.3	80	40
Pinbone, broiled, trimmed of fat (3 oz. piece)	204	0	10.6	5.1	77	62
Pinbone in, broiled (9.9 oz./yield of 1 lb. raw)	1368	0	126.2	60.6	264	131
Pinbone in, broiled, trimmed of fat (5.5 oz./yield of 1 lb. raw)	372	0	19.4	9.3	141	113
Round-bone, broiled (3 oz. piece)	329	0	27.2	13.1	80	48
Round-bone, broiled, trimmed of fat (3 oz. piece)	176	0	6.5	3.1	77	67
Round-bone in, broiled (10.9 oz./yield of 1 lb. raw)	1192	0	98.6	47.3	290	173
Round-bone in, broiled, trimmed of fat (7.2 oz./yield of 1 lb. raw)	420	0	15.6	7.5	185	160
■Sweetbreads, braised (3 oz.)	272	0	19.7	5.1	396	98
T-bone steak, broiled (10.4 oz./yield of 1 lb. raw)	1395	0	127.4	61.2	277	141
T-bone steak, broiled (3 oz. piece)	402	0	36.8	17.6	80	41
T-bone steak, broiled, trimmed of fat (5.8 oz./yield of 1 lb. raw)	368	0	17.0	8.2	150	122
T-bone steak, broiled, trimmed of fat (3 oz. piece)	190	0	8.8	4.2	77	63
Tongue, braised (4 oz.)	277	0.5	18.9	9.1	107	69
LAMB						
Leg, bone in, roasted (9.4 oz./yield of 1 lb. raw)	745	0	50.5	28.3	262	165

Alerts: ● Sodium ★ Sugar ■ Cholesterol

Food Description	Calories	Carbohydrates (grams)	Fat (grams)	Saturated Fat (grams)	Cholesterol (milligrams)	Sodium (milligrams)
Leg, bone in, roasted, trimmed of fat (7.8 oz./yield of 1 lb. raw)	411	0	15.5	8.7	221	155
Leg, boneless, roasted (11.2 oz./yield of 1 lb. raw)	887	0	60.1	33.6	312	197
Leg, boneless, roasted, trimmed of fat (9.3 oz./yield of 1 lb. raw)	491	0	18.5	10.4	264	185
■ Liver, broiled (1.6 oz. slice)	117	1.3	5.6	1.4	197	38
Loin chops, broiled (10.1 oz./yield of 1 lb. raw)	1023	0	83.8	46.9	279	153
Loin chops, broiled, trimmed of fat (6.9 oz./yield of 1 lb. raw)	368	0	14.7	8.2	196	135
Rib chops, broiled (9.5 oz./yield of 1 lb. raw)	1091	0	95.4	53.4	263	131
Rib chops, broiled, trimmed of fat (6 oz./yield of 1 lb. raw)	361	0	18.0	10.1	171	113
Shoulder, bone in, roasted (9.5 oz./yield of 1 lb. raw)	913	0	73.4	41.1	265	143
Shoulder, bone in, roasted, trimmed of fat (7 oz./yield of 1 lb. raw)	410	0	20.0	11.2	200	131
Shoulder, boneless, roasted (11.2 oz./yield of 1 lb. raw)	1075	0	86.5	48.4	312	169
Shoulder, boneless, roasted, trimmed of fat (8.3 oz./yield of 1 lb. raw)	482	0	23.5	13.2	235	154
■ Sweetbreads, braised (3 oz.)	149	0	5.2	1.7	396	98
Tongue, braised (4 oz.)	288	0.6	20.7	11.4	114	67
PORK						
● Bacon, Canadian, broiled or fried, drained (yield from 6 oz. uncooked)	345	0.4	22.0	7.9	105	3219
● Bacon, Canadian style, *Eckrich* (1.2 oz. slice)	60	2.0	2.0	NA	NA	NA
●■ Bacon, cooked, drained (2 medium slices)	89	0.5	7.8	2.5	13	153
●■ Bacon, cooked, drained (2 thick slices)	143	0.8	12.5	4.0	21	245
●■ Bacon, cooked, drained (2 thin slices)	59	0.3	5.2	1.7	9	102
●■ Bacon, cooked, *Oscar Meyer* (1 slice)	35	0.1	3.1	1.1	5	114

Alerts: ● Sodium ★ Sugar ■ Cholesterol

Food Description	Calories	Carbohydrates (grams)	Fat (grams)	Saturated Fat (grams)	Cholesterol (milligrams)	Sodium (milligrams)
Boston Butt						
Bone in, roasted (10.2 oz./yield of 1 lb. raw)	1024	0	82.6	29.8	258	159
Bone in, roasted, trimmed of fat (8.1 oz./yield of 1 lb. raw)	559	0	32.7	11.8	202	151
Boneless, roasted (10.9 oz./yield of 1 lb. raw)	1087	0	87.8	31.6	274	169
Boneless, roasted, trimmed of fat (8.6 oz./yield of 1 lb. raw)	595	0	34.9	12.6	215	161
●Light cure, baked (3 oz. piece)	281	0	21.8	7.9	76	696
●Light cure, baked, trimmed of fat (3 oz. piece)	207	0	11.7	4.2	75	845
●Light cure, bone in, baked, trimmed of fat (9.1 oz./yield of 1 lb. unbaked)	629	0	35.7	12.9	228	2577
●Light cure, boneless, baked (11.8 oz./yield of 1 lb. unbaked)	1109	0	86.4	31.1	299	2754
●Light cure, boneless, baked, trimmed of fat (9.8 oz./yield of 1 lb. unbaked)	678	0	38.5	13.9	246	2776
●Light cure, with bone and skin, baked (11 oz./yield of 1 lb. unbaked)	1030	0	80.2	28.9	278	2557
Roasted (3 oz. slice)	300	0	24.2	8.7	76	46
Roasted, trimmed of fat (3 oz. slice)	207	0	12.2	4.4	75	56
●Breakfast strips, *Lean 'n Tasty* (1 strip)	45	0.2	3.5	1.3	10	220
Ham						
●Country cure, unbaked, relatively lean (1 lb.)	1209	1.2	97.5	35.1	242	3894
●Cured, canned (3 oz. slice)	164	0.8	10.5	3.8	75	797
Fresh, baked (3 oz. slice)	318	0	26.0	9.4	76	47
Fresh, baked, trimmed of fat (3 oz. slice)	184	0	8.5	3.1	75	61
Fresh, boneless, baked (10.9 oz./yield of 1 lb. raw)	1152	0	94.2	33.9	274	173
Fresh, boneless, baked, trimmed of fat (8.1 oz./yield of 1 lb. raw)	495	0	22.8	8.2	201	166

Alerts: ● Sodium ★ Sugar ■ Cholesterol

Food Description	Calories	Carbohydrates (grams)	Fat (grams)	Saturated Fat (grams)	Cholesterol (milligrams)	Sodium (milligrams)
Fresh, with bone and skin, baked (9.2 oz./yield of 1 lb. raw)	980	0	80.2	28.9	233	147
Fresh, with bone and skin, baked, trimmed of fat (6.8 oz./yield of 1 lb. raw)	421	0	19.4	7.0	171	141
•Light cure, baked (3 oz. slice)	246	0	18.8	6.8	76	636
•Light cure, baked, diced (1 cup)	405	0	30.9	11.1	125	1047
•Light cure, baked, ground (1 cup)	318	0	24.3	8.8	98	823
•Light cure, baked, trimmed of fat (3 oz. piece)	159	0	7.5	2.3	75	769
•Light cure, baked, trimmed of fat, diced (1 cup)	262	0	12.3	4.4	123	1268
•Light cure, baked, trimmed of fat, ground (1 cup)	206	0	9.7	3.5	97	996
•Light cure, boneless, baked (13.1 oz./yield of 1 lb. unbaked)	1075	0	82.2	29.6	331	2783
•Light cure, boneless, baked, trimmed of fat (10.2 oz./yield of 1 lb. unbaked)	539	0	25.3	9.1	253	2608
•Light cure, with bone and skin, baked (11.3 oz./yield of 1 lb. unbaked)	925	0	70.7	25.5	285	2394
•Light cure, with bone and skin, baked, trimmed of fat (8.7 oz./yield of 1 lb. unbaked)	460	0	21.6	7.8	216	2228
■Heart, braised, diced (1 cup)	283	0.4	10.0	4.4	397	94
■Liver, fried (3 oz. slice)	205	2.1	9.8	2.9	372	94
Loin						
Chops, bone in, broiled (8.2 oz./yield of 1 lb. raw)	911	0	73.9	26.6	207	141
Chops, bone in, broiled, trimmed of fat (5.9 oz./yield of 1 lb. raw)	454	0	25.9	9.3	148	126
Chops, butterfly, broiled (10.4 oz./yield of 1 lb. raw)	1153	0	93.5	33.7	263	178
Chops, butterfly, broiled, trimmed of fat (7.5 oz./yield of 1 lb. raw)	572	0	32.6	11.7	187	159

Alerts: • Sodium ★ Sugar ■ Cholesterol

Food Description	Calories	Carbohydrates (grams)	Fat (grams)	Saturated Fat (grams)	Cholesterol (milligrams)	Sodium (milligrams)
Roast, bone in, roasted (8.6 oz./yield of 1 lb. raw)	883	0	69.5	25.0	217	146
Roast, bone in, roasted, trimmed of fat (6.9 oz./yield from 1 lb. raw)	495	0	27.7	10.0	172	140
Roast, boneless, roasted (10.9 oz./yield of 1 lb. raw)	1115	0	87.8	31.6	274	184
Roast, boneless, roasted, trimmed of fat (8.7 oz./yield of 1 lb. raw)	627	0	35.1	12.6	217	177
Roast, roasted (3 oz. slice)	308	0	24.2	8.7	76	51
Roast, roasted, trimmed of fat (3 oz. piece)	216	0	12.1	4.3	75	61
Picnic						
• Ham, light cure, baked (3 oz. piece)	275	0	21.4	7.7	76	681
• Ham, light cure, baked, diced (1 cup)	452	0	35.3	12.7	125	1122
• Ham, light cure, baked, ground (1 cup)	335	0	27.7	10.0	98	882
• Ham, light cure, baked, trimmed of fat (3 oz. piece)	179	0	8.4	3.0	75	864
• Ham, light cure, baked, trimmed of fat, diced (1 cup)	295	0	13.9	5.0	123	1423
• Ham, light cure, baked, trimmed of fat, ground (1 cup)	232	0	10.9	3.9	97	1118
• Ham, light cure, boneless, baked (11.8 oz./yield of 1 lb. unbaked)	1085	0	84.7	30.5	299	2694
• Ham, light cure, boneless, baked, trimmed of fat (8.3 oz./yield of 1 lb. unbaked)	496	0	23.3	8.4	207	2389
• Ham, light cure, with bone and skin, baked (9.7 oz./yield of 1 lb. unbaked)	888	0	69.3	24.9	245	2205
• Ham, light cure, with bone and skin, baked, trimmed of fat (6.8 oz./yield of 1 lb. unbaked)	405	0	19.0	6.8	169	1952
Shoulder, fresh, bone in, simmered (8.4 oz./yield of 1 lb.)	890	0	72.6	26.1	212	96

Alerts: • Sodium ★ Sugar ■ Cholesterol

Food Description	Calories	Carbohydrates (grams)	Fat (grams)	Saturated Fat (grams)	Cholesterol (milligrams)	Sodium (milligrams)
Shoulder, fresh, bone in, simmered, trimmed of fat (6.2 oz./yield of 1 lb. raw)	373	0	17.2	6.2	155	89
Shoulder, fresh, boneless, simmered (10.2 oz./yield of 1 lb.)	1085	0	88.4	31.8	258	117
Shoulder, fresh, boneless, simmered, trimmed of fat (7.6 oz./yield of 1 lb. raw)	456	0	21.1	7.6	189	109
Shoulder, fresh, simmered (3 oz. slice)	318	0	25.9	9.3	76	34
Shoulder, fresh, simmered, trimmed of fat (3 oz. slice)	180	0	8.3	3.0	75	43
Pig's feet, pickled (2 oz.)	113	0	8.4	3.0	51	39
Spareribs, braised (6.3 oz./yield of 1 lb. raw)	792	0	70.0	25.2	160	65
Tongue, braised (4 oz.)	287	0.6	19.7	6.8	100	69

VEAL

Food Description	Calories	Carbohydrates (grams)	Fat (grams)	Saturated Fat (grams)	Cholesterol (milligrams)	Sodium (milligrams)
Breast, bone in, braised or stewed (8.2 oz./yield of 1 lb. raw)	718	0	50.2	24.1	239	108
Breast, boneless, braised or stewed (10.6 oz./yield of 1 lb. raw)	906	0	63.4	30.4	302	136
Chuck stew meat, cooked (10.6 oz./yield of 1 lb. raw)	703	0	38.3	18.4	302	145
Cutlets, boneless, braised (11.3 oz./yield of 1 lb. raw)	693	0	35.6	17.1	324	213
Cutlet, boneless, braised (3 oz.)	184	0	9.4	4.5	86	56
■Heart (calf), braised, diced (1 cup)	302	2.6	13.2	7.3	397	163
■Liver (calf), fried (3 oz. slice)	222	3.4	11.2	2.6	372	100
Loin, bone in, braised or broiled (9.5 oz./yield of 1 lb. raw)	629	0	36.0	17.3	272	174
Loin, boneless, braised or broiled (11.4 oz./yield of 1 lb. raw)	758	0	43.4	20.8	327	209
Loin, cooked (3 oz. slice)	199	0	11.4	5.5	86	55
Rib roast, bone in, roasted (8.5 oz./yield of 1 lb. raw)	648	0	40.7	19.6	243	160
Rib roast, boneless, roasted (11 oz./yield of 1 lb. raw)	842	0	52.9	25.4	316	208
Rib roast, roasted (3 oz. slice)	229	0	14.4	6.9	86	56

Alerts: ● Sodium ★ Sugar ■ Cholesterol

Food Description	Calories	Carbohydrates (grams)	Fat (grams)	Saturated Fat (grams)	Cholesterol (milligrams)	Sodium (milligrams)
Round roast, bone in, roasted (8.7 oz./yield of 1 lb. raw)	534	0	27.4	13.2	249	164
Round roast, cooked (3 oz. slice)	184	0	9.4	4.5	86	56
■Sweetbreads (calf), braised (3 oz.)	143	0	2.7	0.9	396	98
Tongue (calf), braised (4 oz.)	182	1.1	6.8	3.4	112	69

Nuts and Seeds

Food Description	Calories	Carbohydrates (grams)	Fat (grams)	Saturated Fat (grams)	Cholesterol (milligrams)	Sodium (milligrams)
●★Filling, almond, *Solo* (1 oz.)	73	13.1	1.9	NA	0	2
●★Filling, nut, *Solo* (1 oz.)	86	11.4	4.1	NA	0	19
●★Filling, pecan, *Solo* (1 oz.)	93	11.6	4.8	NA	0	18
●★Filling, poppy, *Solo* (1 oz.)	83	14.0	2.4	NA	0	13
Peanut Butter						
●★Creamy, *Jif* (2 Tbsp.)	190	6.0	16.0	3.0	0	155
●★Creamy, *Planters* (2 Tbsp.)	190	6.0	16.0	3.0	0	190
●★Creamy, *Skippy* (2 Tbsp.)	190	5.0	17.0	3.0	0	150
●★Crunchy, *Jif* (2 Tbsp.)	190	6.0	16.0	3.0	0	130
●★Grape combination, *Goobers, Smucker's* (2 oz.)	250	28.0	12.0	1.0	0	154
★Low sodium, *Featherweight* (2 Tbsp.)	180	4.0	15.0	NA	0	5
★Low sodium, *Nutradiet* (1 Tbsp.)	93	2.0	8.0	NA	0	10
●★Super chunk, old fashioned, *Skippy* (2 Tbsp.)	190	5.0	16.0	2.0	0	150
Seeds, pumpkin (1 cup)	774	21.0	65.4	11.8	0	0
Seeds, sesame (1 cup)	873	26.4	80.1	11.2	0	90
Seeds, sunflower, hulled (1 cup)	812	28.9	68.6	8.2	0	43
NUTS						
Almond meal, partly defatted (1 oz.)	116	8.2	5.2	0.4	0	2
Almonds, dried, shelled, slivered, packed (1 cup)	807	26.3	73.2	5.9	0	5
●Almonds, dry roasted, *Planters* (1 oz.)	170	6.0	15.0	2.0	0	220

Alerts: ● Sodium ★ Sugar ■ Cholesterol

Food Description	Calories	Carbohydrates (grams)	Fat (grams)	Saturated Fat (grams)	Cholesterol (milligrams)	Sodium (milligrams)
• Almonds, roasted in oil, salted (1 oz.)	178	5.5	16.4	1.3	0	56
Brazil, shelled (1 cup)	916	15.3	93.7	18.7	0	1
Butternuts, in shell (1 lb.)	399	5.3	38.9	3.2	0	1
• Cashews, dry roasted, *Planters* (1 oz.)	160	9.0	13.0	3.0	0	220
• Cashews, salted, *Planters* (1 oz.)	170	8.0	14.0	3.0	0	220
Cashews, unsalted, *Planters* (1 oz.)	160	9.0	13.0	3.0	0	10
Chestnuts, in shell (10 nuts)	141	30.7	1.1	0	0	30
Coconut meat (2" square piece)	156	4.2	15.9	13.7	0	10
Filberts (10 nuts)	87	2.3	8.6	0.4	0	Tr.
Filberts, shelled, chopped (1 cup)	729	19.2	71.8	3.6	0	2
Lychees (10 nuts)	58	14.8	0.3	0	0	3
• Mixed, dry roasted, *Planters* (1 oz.)	160	7.0	14.0	2.0	0	220
• Mixed, *Planters* (1 oz.)	180	6.0	16.0	3.0	0	220
Mixed, unsalted, *Planters* (1 oz.)	170	7.0	15.0	2.0	0	10
• Peanuts, dry roasted, *Planters* (1 oz.)	160	6.0	14.0	2.0	0	220
• Peanuts, Spanish, *Planters* (1 oz.)	170	5.0	15.0	5.0	0	220
Peanuts, unsalted, *Planters* (1 oz.)	170	5.5	15.0	2.0	0	10
Pecans (10 medium)	277	5.9	28.7	2.0	0	0
Pecans, chopped (1 cup)	811	17.2	84.0	5.9	0	0
Piñons, shelled (1 oz.)	180	5.8	17.2	0.9	0	Tr.
Pistachios, in shell (1 lb.)	1347	43.0	121.8	12.2	0	2
• Soy, *Planters* (1 oz.)	130	10.0	7.0	1.0	0	220
Sunflower, unsalted, *Planters* (1 oz.)	170	5.0	15.0	2.0	0	10
Walnuts, black, shelled (1 oz.)	178	4.2	16.8	1.0	0	1
Walnuts, English or Persian, chopped (1 cup)	781	19.0	76.8	5.4	0	2
Walnuts, halves and pieces, *Diamond* (1 cup)	679	12.8	66.3	NA	0	NA

Alerts: • Sodium ★ Sugar ■ Cholesterol

Pancakes and Waffles

Food Description	Calories	Carbohydrates (grams)	Fat (grams)	Saturated Fat (grams)	Cholesterol (milligrams)	Sodium (milligrams)
Pancake and Waffle Mix						
●★Buckwheat, dry (1 cup)	426	91.4	2.5	0	0	1734
●★Buckwheat, dry, *Aunt Jemima* (¼ cup)	107	21.3	0.8	0	0	429
●★Buttermilk, complete, dry, *Aunt Jemima* (⅓ cup)	236	46.2	2.3	NA	NA	NA
●★Buttermilk, complete, dry, *General Mills* (½ cup)	210	41.0	3.0	NA	NA	580
●★Buttermilk, complete, *Hungry Jack* (3 4″ cakes)	180	35.0	3.0	NA	NA	675
●★Buttermilk, dry, *Aunt Jemima* (⅓ cup)	175	36.5	0.7	0	NA	847
●★Buttermilk, dry, *General Mills* (⅓ cup)	170	36.0	1.0	0	0	755
●★Buttermilk, dry, *Log Cabin* (mix for 3 4″ cakes)	140	31.0	0	0	NA	645
●★Buttermilk, dry, *Hungry Jack* (mix for 3 4″ cakes)	130	27.0	1.0	0	NA	540
★Low cholesterol, sugar restricted, prepared, *Sweet 'N Low* (4 pancakes)	140	23.0	5.0	NA	5	40
★No salt, prepared, *Featherweight* (3 pancakes)	130	24.0	1.0	NA	0	70
●★Original, dry, *Aunt Jemima* (¼ cup)	108	22.5	0.6	0	0	482
●★Plain or buttermilk, dry (1 cup)	481	102.2	2.4	0	0	1934
●★Regular, complete, *Log Cabin* (3 4″ cakes)	180	33.0	3.0	NA	NA	605
●★Regular, dry, *Hungry Jack Extra Lights* (mix for 3 4″ cakes)	110	25.0	0	0	0	450
●★Regular, dry, *Log Cabin* (mix for 3 4″ cakes)	110	23.0	0	0	0	475
●★Whole wheat, dry, *Aunt Jemima* (⅓ cup)	142	28.5	0.5	0	0	NA
●★Pancake batter, frozen, *Aunt Jemima* (3 4″ pancakes)	210	42.2	1.6	NA	NA	NA

Alerts: ● Sodium ★ Sugar ■ Cholesterol

Food Description	Calories	Carbohydrates (grams)	Fat (grams)	Saturated Fat (grams)	Cholesterol (milligrams)	Sodium (milligrams)
•★ Pancake batter, frozen, blueberry, *Aunt Jemima* (3 4″ pancakes)	205	41.5	1.6	NA	NA	NA
•★ Pancakes, frozen, whipped maple topping, *Hungry Jack Microwave Pancakes* (4 pancakes)	370	55.0	15.0	NA	NA	640
•★■ Pancakes, homemade (6″ cake)	169	24.9	5.1	1.3	39	310
Waffles						
•★■ Blueberry, frozen, *Aunt Jemima* (1.25 oz. waffle)	86	13.6	2.5	NA	NA	667
•★■ Blueberry, frozen, *Downyflake* (2 waffles)	180	32.0	4.0	NA	NA	NA
•★■ Blueberry, frozen, *Eggo* (1 waffle)	130	18.0	5.0	NA	NA	260
•★■ Butter flavor, frozen, *Downyflake* (2 waffles)	130	22.0	5.0	NA	NA	NA
•★■ Buttermilk, frozen, *Aunt Jemima* (1 jumbo)	86	13.6	2.5	NA	NA	357
•★■ Buttermilk, frozen, *Downyflake* (2 waffles)	170	30.0	4.0	NA	NA	NA
•★■ Frozen (1 large)	86	14.3	2.1	0.5	43	219
•★■ Frozen, *Downyflake* (2 waffles)	120	20.0	3.0	NA	NA	465
•★■ Homemade (7″ round)	209	28.1	7.3	2.4	94	356
•★■ Homestyle, frozen, *Eggo* (1 waffle)	120	17.0	5.0	NA	NA	265
•★■ Original, frozen, *Aunt Jemima* (1 jumbo)	86	13.6	2.5	NA	NA	349
•★■ Strawberry, frozen, *Eggo* (1 waffle)	130	18.0	5.0	NA	NA	265

Pasta and Pasta Dishes

	Calories	Carbohydrates (grams)	Fat (grams)	Saturated Fat (grams)	Cholesterol (milligrams)	Sodium (milligrams)
Dumplings, dry, *Mueller* (2 oz.)	210	41.0	1.0	0	0	NA
Lasagna, curly, dry, *Prince* (2 oz.)	204	40.0	1.8	0	0	1

Alerts: • Sodium ★ Sugar ■ Cholesterol

Food Description	Calories	Carbohydrates (grams)	Fat (grams)	Saturated Fat (grams)	Cholesterol (milligrams)	Sodium (milligrams)
Lasagna, dry, *Creamette* (2 oz.)	210	41.0	1.0	0	0	NA
Macaroni, all shapes, dry, *Mueller's* (2 oz.)	210	41.0	1.0	0	0	9
Macaroni, cooked without salt, firm (4.4 cups)	844	171.6	2.8	0	0	6
Macaroni, cooked without salt, soft (5⅓ cups)	821	170.2	3.0	0	0	7
Macaroni, dry (8 oz.)	838	170.7	2.7	0	0	4
Macaroni, dry, *American Beauty* (2 oz.)	210	41.0	1.0	0	0	5
Macaroni, dry, *Creamette* (2 oz.)	210	41.0	1.0	0	0	NA
Macaroni, elbo, dry, *Foulds* (2 oz.)	210	41.0	1.0	0	0	1
Mostaccioli, dry, *La Rosa* (2 oz.)	210	41.0	1.0	1.0	NA	NA
Mostaccioli, dry, *Prince* (2 oz.)	204	40.0	1.8	0	0	1
● Mostaccioli, lined, dry, *Prince Superoni* (2 oz.)	210	36.0	2.0	NA	NA	45
Mostaccioli rigata, dry, *Ravarino and Freschi* (2 oz.)	210	41.0	1.0	0	0	NA
Noodles						
● Chow mein, canned (1 cup)	220	26.1	10.6	2.7	5	450
■ Egg, bows, dry, *Prince* (2 oz.)	220	40.0	3.0	NA	NA	12
■ Egg, dry (8 oz.)	881	163.4	10.4	3.3	213	11
■ Egg, dry, *American Beauty* (2 oz.)	220	40.0	3.0	NA	NA	5
■ Egg, dry, *Dutch Mill* (2 oz.)	220	40.0	3.0	0	NA	4
■ Egg, dry, *Greenfield* (2 oz.)	210	37.0	3.0	NA	NA	Tr.
■ Egg, dry, *Mrs. Grass* (2 oz.)	220	40.0	3.0	NA	NA	NA
■ Egg, dry, *Mueller* (2 oz.)	220	40.0	3.0	0	NA	NA
■ Egg, flakes, dry, *Streit's* (2 oz.)	220	40.0	3.0	0	NA	5
■ Egg, premium, no salt, dry, *Manischewitz* (2 oz.)	220	40.0	3.0	NA	NA	4
● Egg substitute, cholesterol free, dry, *No Yolks* (2 oz.)	210	40.0	2.0	NA	0	50
■ Spinach, dry, *La Rosa* (2 oz.)	220	40.0	3.0	NA	NA	NA
Rotini, dry, *Prince* (2 oz.)	204	40.0	1.8	0	0	1
Shells, dry, *American Beauty* (2 oz.)	210	41.0	1.0	0	0	5
Shells, dry, *La Rosa* (2 oz.)	210	41.0	1.0	NA	NA	NA
Shells, for filling, dry, *Prince Superoni* (2 oz.)	210	42.0	1.0	0	0	1

Alerts: ● Sodium ★ Sugar ■ Cholesterol

Food Description	Calories	Carbohydrates (grams)	Fat (grams)	Saturated Fat (grams)	Cholesterol (milligrams)	Sodium (milligrams)
Shells, medium, dry, *Prince* (2 oz.)	204	40.0	1.8	0	0	1
Spaghetti						
All shapes, dry, *Mueller's* (2 oz.)	210	41.0	1.0	0	0	9
Cooked, firm (4.4 cups)	884	171.6	2.8	0	0	6
Cooked, soft (5⅓ cups)	821	170.2	3.0	0	0	7
Dry (8 oz.)	838	170.7	2.7	0	0	4
Dry, *American Beauty* (2 oz.)	210	41.0	1.0	0	0	5
Dry, *Creamette* (2 oz.)	210	41.0	1.0	0	0	NA
Dry, *Foulds* (2 oz.)	210	41.0	1.0	0	0	2
Dry, *La Rosa* (2 oz.)	210	41.0	1.0	NA	NA	NA
Dry, *Red Cross* (2 oz.)	210	41.0	1.0	0	0	NA
Thin, dry, *Prince* (2 oz.)	204	40.0	1.8	0	0	1
● Thin, dry, *Prince Superoni* (2 oz.)	210	36.0	2.0	0	0	45
Vermicelli, dry, *Prince* (2 oz.)	204	40.0	1.8	0	0	1
PASTA DISHES						
●★ Lasagna, dry, *Stir-N-Serv, Golden Grain* (1.4 oz.)	140	26.0	3.0	NA	NA	NA
●★■ Lasagna, with meat sauce, frozen, *Green Giant* (3½ oz.)	116	12.6	7.6	NA	NA	488
●★■ Lasagna, with meat sauce, frozen, *Swanson* (11¾ oz.)	450	46.0	18.0	NA	NA	1130
●★■ Lasagna, with meat sauce, frozen, *Swanson Hungry-Man* (12¾ oz.)	540	51.0	28.0	NA	NA	1070
Macaroni and Cheese						
● Casserole, frozen, *Morton* (8 oz.)	270	36.0	9.0	NA	24	900
●■ Frozen, *Green Giant* (3½ oz.)	126	13.9	5.4	NA	NA	519
●■ Frozen, *Stouffers* (6 oz.)	260	24.0	12.0	NA	NA	780
●■ Frozen, *Swanson* (12 oz.)	420	40.0	21.0	NA	NA	1470
●■ Homemade with butter (1 cup)	430	40.2	22.2	11.9	68	1086
●■ Homemade with margarine (1 cup)	430	40.2	22.2	8.9	42	1086
●■ Mix, deluxe, *Kraft* (⅕ box)	250	34.0	8.0	4.0	18	595
●■ *Mug-O-Lunch* (1 pouch)	240	41.0	5.0	NA	NA	695
●■ Pie, frozen, *Swanson* (8 oz.)	230	26.0	10.0	NA	NA	655
● Spiral, mix, *Kraft* (¼ box)	170	30.0	2.0	1.0	0	355
● Twists and cheddar dinner, dry, *Prince* (1.8 oz.)	190	36.0	1.9	NA	NA	413
●★ Macaroni with beef and tomato sauce, canned, *Beefy Mac, Franco-American* (7½ oz.)	220	28.0	8.0	NA	NA	1235

Alerts: ● Sodium ★ Sugar ■ Cholesterol

Food Description	Calories	Carbohydrates (grams)	Fat (grams)	Saturated Fat (grams)	Cholesterol (milligrams)	Sodium (milligrams)
•★Macaroni, with beef and tomato sauce, canned, *Beefy O's, Franco-American* (7½ oz.)	220	30.0	8.0	NA	NA	1235
•★Macaroni, with beef and tomato sauce, frozen, *Green Giant* (3½ oz.)	91	12.0	2.8	NA	NA	250
Noodles						
•■Almondine, dry, *Side Quick* (¼ package)	170	25.0	5.0	NA	NA	700
• Beef flavor sauce, dry, *Mug-O-Lunch* (1 pouch)	170	30.0	3.0	NA	NA	825
•■Egg, with beef sauce, mix, *Betty Crocker Side Quicks* (¼ package)	120	21.0	2.0	NA	NA	NA
•■Egg, with cheese sauce, mix, *Betty Crocker Side Quicks* (¼ package)	120	21.0	2.0	NA	NA	NA
•■Egg, with chicken, mix, *Kraft* (¼ box)	190	30.0	4.0	1.0	65	815
•■Parmesan, dry, *Noodle Roni* (1.2 oz.)	130	23.0	2.0	NA	NA	NA
•■Romanoff, mix, *Betty Crocker* (¼ package)	170	22.0	6.0	NA	NA	580
•■Stroganoff, mix, *Betty Crocker* (¼ package)	150	24.0	4.0	NA	NA	480
•★Ravioli, in beef sauce, canned, *Featherweight* (8 oz.)	230	35.0	6.0	NA	NA	100
•★Ravioli, with beef and tomato sauce, canned, *Franco-American Raviolio's* (7¾ oz.)	220	33.0	6.0	NA	NA	925
•★Ravioli, with cheese and tomato sauce, canned, *Franco-American Raviolios* (7½ oz.)	260	39.0	8.0	NA	NA	975
•★Rotini, with meatballs and tomato sauce, canned, *Franco-American* (7⅜ oz.)	180	24.0	7.0	NA	NA	885
• Shells and cheddar dinner, dry, *Prince* (1.8 oz.)	190	36.0	1.9	NA	NA	413
Spaghetti						
•★Casserole, with meat, frozen, *Morton* (8 oz.)	220	31.0	6.0	NA	25	760
• Dinner, dry, *Kraft* (¼ package)	200	37.0	2.0	1.0	0	735

Alerts: • Sodium ★ Sugar ■ Cholesterol

Food Description	Calories	Carbohydrates (grams)	Fat (grams)	Saturated Fat (grams)	Cholesterol (milligrams)	Sodium (milligrams)
●★With meatballs and sauce, canned, *Featherweight* (7½ oz.)	200	28.0	5.0	NA	NA	95
●★With meatballs and tomato sauce, canned, *Franco-American* (7⅜ oz.)	210	24.0	9.0	NA	NA	945
●★With meatballs and tomato sauce, canned, *Spaghetti O's, Franco-American* (7¼ oz.)	210	24.0	9.0	NA	NA	1125
●★With meatballs and tomato sauce, frozen, *Green Giant* (3½ oz.)	105	11.4	5.2	NA	NA	475
●★With meatballs, frozen, *Morton* (11 oz.)	360	61.0	8.0	NA	27	905
●★With meat sauce, canned, *Franco-American* (7½ oz.)	220	26.0	10.0	NA	NA	1105
●★With meat sauce, frozen, *Banquet* (8 oz.)	311	31.3	14.5	NA	NA	1426
●★With meat sauce, frozen, *Stouffers* (14 oz.)	445	62.0	12.0	NA	NA	1970
●★With meat sauce, mix, *Kraft* (⅕ box)	230	31.0	8.0	2.0	10	595
●★With tomato sauce and cheese, canned, *Franco-American* (7⅜ oz.)	170	33.0	2.0	NA	NA	820
●★With tomato sauce and cheese, homemade (1 cup)	260	37.0	8.8	2.0	8	955
●★■With tomato sauce, meatballs and cheese, homemade (1 cup)	332	38.7	11.7	3.3	74	1009

Pies and Pastries

PASTRIES						
●★Bun, caramel, frozen, *Sara Lee* (1 bun)	116	15.2	5.4	NA	NA	111

Alerts: ● Sodium ★ Sugar ■ Cholesterol

Food Description	Calories	Carbohydrates (grams)	Fat (grams)	Saturated Fat (grams)	Cholesterol (milligrams)	Sodium (milligrams)
●★Bun, honey, frozen, *Morton* (2.3 oz.)	230	31.0	11.0	NA	1	150
●★■Bun, honey, *Hostess* (4¾ oz.)	580	63.0	34.0	NA	31	835
Coffee Cake						
●★■Almond, frozen, *Sara Lee* (⅛ cake)	164	20.1	8.0	NA	NA	158
●★Apple cinnamon, mix, *Pillsbury* (⅛ package)	210	39.0	5.0	NA	0	140
●★■Apple, frozen, *Sara Lee* (⅛ cake)	174	24.1	7.6	NA	NA	208
●★Butter pecan, mix, *Pillsbury* (⅛ package)	220	38.0	6.0	NA	0	225
●★■Butter streusel, frozen, *Sara Lee* (⅛ cake)	164	20.3	8.0	NA	NA	179
●★■Cinnamon streusel, frozen, *Sara Lee* (⅛ cake)	154	19.0	7.7	NA	NA	156
●★Mix, *Aunt Jemima* (1.3 oz.)	162	28.7	4.4	NA	0	226
●★■Pecan, frozen, *Sara Lee* (⅛ cake)	153	19.1	8.6	NA	NA	159
●★Sour cream, mix, *Pillsbury* (⅛ package)	240	34.0	10.0	NA	0	210
●★■Coffee ring, maple crunch, frozen, *Sara Lee* (⅛ ring)	138	17.2	6.7	NA	NA	131
●★■Coffee ring, raspberry, frozen, *Sara Lee* (⅛ ring)	133	18.5	5.8	NA	NA	120
●★■Cream puff, custard filled (4.6 oz.)	303	26.6	18.1	5.6	187	107
●★■Cream puff, vanilla, frozen, *Rich's* (1 cream puff)	167	23.4	7.2	NA	40	117
●★■Danish (1.5 oz. piece)	127	19.2	9.9	2.9	27	153
●★■Danish, caramel nut, *Pillsbury* (2 rolls)	300	39.0	15.0	NA	NA	485
●★■Danish, cheese, frozen, *Sara Lee* (1 roll)	131	13.9	7.2	NA	NA	125
●★■Danish, cinnamon raisin, frozen, *Sara Lee* (1 roll)	147	17.3	7.6	NA	NA	132
●★■Danish, cinnamon raisin, iced, *Pillsbury* (2 rolls)	270	40.0	11.0	NA	NA	450
●★■Danish, pecan, frozen, *Sara Lee* (1 roll)	148	18.3	7.3	NA	NA	119
Doughnuts						
●★Bavarian creme, frozen, *Morton* (2 oz.)	180	22.0	9.0	NA	11	75
●★Boston creme, frozen, *Morton* (2⅓ oz.)	210	28.0	9.0	NA	11	90

Alerts: ● Sodium ★ Sugar ■ Cholesterol

Food Description	Calories	Carbohydrates (grams)	Fat (grams)	Saturated Fat (grams)	Cholesterol (milligrams)	Sodium (milligrams)
●★■ Cake (⅞ oz.)	98	12.8	4.7	1.2	15	125
●★ Chocolate iced, frozen, *Morton* (1.5 oz.)	150	20.0	7.0	NA	10	75
●★ Cinnamon, *Hostess* (1 oz.)	110	15.0	6.0	NA	6	110
●★ Crunch, *Hostess* (1 oz.)	100	16.0	4.0	NA	4	105
●★ Glazed, frozen, *Morton* (1.5 oz.)	150	19.0	7.0	NA	10	75
●★ Holes, devil's food, frozen, *Morton* (1.6 oz.)	160	22.0	8.0	NA	5	105
●★ Holes, honey wheat, frozen, *Morton* (1.6 oz.)	160	21.0	8.0	NA	5	140
●★ Holes, vanilla, frozen, *Morton* (1.6 oz.)	160	22.0	8.0	NA	5	123
●★ Jelly, frozen, *Morton* (1.8 oz.)	180	23.0	8.0	NA	11	75
●★ Old fashioned, *Hostess* (1.5 oz.)	170	20.0	10.0	NA	9	150
●★ Plain, *Hostess* (1 oz.)	110	12.0	7.0	NA	7	135
●★ Powdered sugar, *Hostess* (1 oz.)	110	15.0	6.0	NA	6	110
●★■ Dumpling, apple, *Pepperidge Farm* (1 dumpling)	280	31.0	17.0	NA	NA	206
●★■ Eclair, cream filled, chocolate covered, frozen, *Rich's* (1 eclair)	220	26.0	12.0	NA	40	75
●★■ Eclair, custard filled, chocolate iced (3.5 oz.)	239	23.2	13.6	4.4	136	82
●★■ Popover, homemade (1 popover)	90	10.3	3.7	1.3	59	88
●★ *Pop-Tart*, blueberry (1 pastry)	210	36.0	6.0	NA	NA	250
●★ *Pop-Tart*, blueberry, frosted (1 pastry)	210	35.0	6.0	NA	NA	235
●★ *Pop-Tart*, brown sugar-cinnamon (1 pastry)	210	32.0	8.0	NA	NA	235
●★ *Pop-Tart*, cherry (1 pastry)	210	37.0	6.0	NA	NA	265
●★ *Pop-Tart*, cherry, frosted (1 pastry)	210	37.0	6.0	NA	NA	235
●★ *Pop-Tart*, chocolate chip, frosted (1 pastry)	210	35.0	6.0	NA	NA	280
●★ *Pop-Tart*, chocolate fudge, frosted (1 pastry)	200	36.0	4.0	NA	NA	255
●★ *Pop-Tart*, chocolate-vanilla cream, frosted (1 pastry)	200	34.0	5.0	NA	NA	260
●★ *Pop-Tart*, concord grape, frosted (1 pastry)	210	36.0	6.0	NA	NA	250

Alerts: ● Sodium ★ Sugar ■ Cholesterol

Food Description	Calories	Carbohydrates (grams)	Fat (grams)	Saturated Fat (grams)	Cholesterol (milligrams)	Sodium (milligrams)
●★*Pop-Tart,* raspberry, frosted (1 pastry)	210	36.0	6.0	NA	NA	255
●★*Pop-Tart,* strawberry (1 pastry)	210	36.0	6.0	NA	NA	270
●★*Pop-Tart,* strawberry, frosted (1 pastry)	210	36.0	6.0	NA	NA	235
●★■ Square, blueberry, *Pepperidge Farm* (1 square)	280	35.0	15.0	NA	NA	188
●★■ Strudel, apple, *Pepperidge Farm* (3 oz.)	250	31.0	13.0	NA	NA	174
●★ Sweet rolls, cinnamon, iced, *Ballard* (2 rolls)	200	34.0	6.0	NA	NA	620
●★ Sweet roll, cinnamon, iced, *Pillsbury* (2 rolls)	230	35.0	8.0	NA	NA	500
●★ Sweet roll, honey, frozen, *Sara Lee* (1 roll)	112	15.2	4.7	NA	NA	119
●★■ Tart, apple, *Pepperidge Farm* (1 tart)	280	33.0	16.0	NA	NA	176
●★■ Tart, blueberry, *Pepperidge Farm* (1 tart)	280	35.0	15.0	NA	NA	188
●★■ Tart, cherry, *Pepperidge Farm* (1 tart)	280	35.0	15.0	NA	NA	196
●★■ Tart, lemon, *Pepperidge Farm* (1 tart)	320	37.0	19.0	NA	NA	218
●★■ Tart, raspberry, *Pepperidge Farm* (1 tart)	320	34.0	19.0	NA	NA	238
●★ Tart, shell, *Pepperidge Farm* (1 shell)	90	10.0	5.0	NA	NA	71
●★ Turnover, apple, *Pillsbury* (1 turnover)	180	22.0	9.0	NA	NA	300
●★■ Turnover, blueberry, *Pepperidge Farm* (1 turnover)	320	32.0	20.0	NA	NA	254
●★ Turnover, cherry, *Pillsbury* (1 turnover)	190	24.0	9.0	NA	NA	300
●★■ Turnover, peach, *Pepperidge Farm* (1 turnover)	320	33.0	20.0	NA	NA	250
●★■ Turnover, raspberry, *Pepperidge Farm* (1 turnover)	340	37.0	20.0	NA	NA	254
PIES						
●★ Apple, frozen (⅙ of 8″ pie)	234	36.8	9.8	2.3	0	196
●★ Apple, frozen, *Morton* (4 oz.)	290	41.0	13.0	NA	12	240
●★ Apple, frozen, *Sara Lee* (⅙ pie)	376	43.2	21.4	NA	NA	279

Alerts: ● Sodium ★ Sugar ■ Cholesterol

Food Description	Calories	Carbohydrates (grams)	Fat (grams)	Saturated Fat (grams)	Cholesterol (milligrams)	Sodium (milligrams)
●★Apple, homemade (⅙ of 9″ pie)	404	60.2	17.5	4.5	0	475
●★Apple, *Hostess* (4½ oz.)	400	54.0	20.0	NA	18	415
●★Banana cream, frozen, *Banquet* (14 oz.)	1032	119.6	57.6	NA	NA	464
●★Banana cream, frozen, *Great Little Dessert, Morton* (3½ oz.)	250	27.0	15.0	NA	15	200
●★■Banana custard, homemade (⅙ of 9″ pie)	336	46.7	14.1	4.5	88	442
●★Berry, *Hostess* (4½ oz.)	400	51.0	20.0	NA	18	410
●★Blackberry, homemade (⅙ of 9″ pie)	384	54.4	17.4	4.3	0	635
●★Blueberry, frozen, *Morton* (4 oz.)	280	39.0	14.0	NA	12	250
●★Blueberry, frozen, *Sara Lee* (⅙ pie)	404	44.8	28.7	NA	NA	220
●★Blueberry, homemade (⅙ of 9″ pie)	382	55.1	17.1	4.2	0	635
●★Blueberry, *Hostess* (4½ oz.)	390	49.0	20.0	NA	18	410
●★■Boston cream, homemade (1/12 of 8″ pie)	208	34.4	6.5	2.0	59	128
●★Boston cream, mix, *Betty Crocker* (⅛ package)	220	46.0	4.0	NA	NA	375
●★■Butterscotch, homemade (⅙ of 9″ pie)	406	58.2	16.7	6.0	79	487
●★Cherry, frozen (⅙ of 8″ pie)	282	43.1	11.6	2.9	0	222
●★Cherry, frozen, *Morton* (4 oz.)	300	42.0	14.0	NA	12	250
●★Cherry, frozen, *Sara Lee* (⅙ pie)	385	48.0	21.2	NA	NA	233
●★Cherry, homemade (⅙ of 9″ pie)	412	60.7	17.9	4.7	0	480
●★Cherry, *Hostess* (4½ oz.)	420	59.0	20.0	NA	18	410
●★■Chocolate chiffon, homemade (⅙ of 9″ pie)	354	47.2	16.5	6.7	151	272
●★Chocolate cream, frozen, *Banquet* (14 oz.)	1064	131.0	54.6	NA	NA	381
●★Chocolate cream, frozen, *Great Little Dessert, Morton* (3½ oz.)	270	29.0	17.0	NA	15	200
●★Chocolate cream, mix, *No Bake Desserts, Pillsbury* (⅙ package)	250	48.0	6.0	NA	NA	330
●★■Chocolate meringue, homemade (⅙ of 9″ pie)	383	50.9	18.2	6.8	85	389

Alerts: ● Sodium ★ Sugar ■ Cholesterol

Food Description	Calories	Carbohydrates (grams)	Fat (grams)	Saturated Fat (grams)	Cholesterol (milligrams)	Sodium (milligrams)
●★ Coconut cream, frozen, Banquet (14 oz.)	1044	114.7	61.3	NA	NA	389
●★ Coconut cream, frozen, Great Little Dessert, Morton (3½ oz.)	270	25.0	19.0	NA	15	190
●★■ Coconut custard, frozen (⅙ of 8" pie)	249	29.5	12.0	5.0	102	252
●★■ Coconut custard, frozen, Great Little Dessert, Morton (6½ oz.)	370	53.0	15.0	NA	110	495
●★■ Coconut custard, homemade (⅙ of 9" pie)	357	37.8	19.0	7.6	155	375
●★ Crust, deep, Pepperidge Farm (¼ crust)	130	10.0	9.0	NA	NA	100
●★ Crust, homemade (1 pie shell)	900	78.8	60.1	14.9	0	1099
●★ Crust, mix (1 cup)	626	59.4	39.2	9.7	0	831
●★ Crust, mix (10 oz.)	1482	140.6	92.9	23.0	0	1968
●★ Crust, mix, Betty Crocker (1/16 package)	120	10.0	8.0	NA	NA	140
●★ Crust, mix, Pillsbury (⅙ of a 2 crust pie)	290	27.0	18.0	NA	NA	400
●★ Crust, Pillsbury, All Ready Pie Crust (⅛ of 2 crust pie)	250	22.0	17.0	NA	NA	370
●★ Crust, sticks, Pillsbury (⅙ of a 2 crust pie)	290	27.0	18.0	NA	NA	400
●★ Crust, top, Pepperidge Farm (¼ top)	190	15.0	14.0	NA	NA	152
●★■ Custard, homemade (⅙ of 9" pie)	331	35.6	16.9	5.7	160	436
●★ Dutch apple, frozen, Great Little Dessert, Morton (7¾ oz.)	600	94.0	23.0	NA	13	470
●★■ Lemon chiffon, homemade (⅙ of 9" pie)	338	47.3	13.6	3.7	183	423
●★ Lemon chiffon mix, No Bake Desserts, Pillsbury (⅙ package)	230	45.0	3.0	NA	NA	320
●★ Lemon cream, frozen, Great Little Dessert, Morton (3½ oz.)	250	27.0	15.0	NA	15	200
●★■ Lemon, Hostess (4½ oz.)	420	53.0	22.0	NA	30	420
●★■ Lemon meringue, homemade (⅙ of 9" pie)	357	52.8	14.3	4.3	130	394
●★ Mince, frozen, Morton (4 oz.)	310	46.0	14.0	NA	12	355

Alerts: ● Sodium ★ Sugar ■ Cholesterol

Food Description	Calories	Carbohydrates (grams)	Fat (grams)	Saturated Fat (grams)	Cholesterol (milligrams)	Sodium (milligrams)
●★ Mince, homemade (⅙ of 9″ pie)	428	65.1	18.2	4.8	2	707
●★ Peach, frozen, *Morton* (4 oz.)	280	39.0	13.0	NA	12	260
●★ Peach, frozen, *Sara Lee* (⅙ pie)	432	56.2	24.6	NA	NA	253
●★ Peach, homemade (⅙ of 9″ pie)	403	60.4	16.9	4.2	0	635
●★ Peach, *Hostess* (4½ oz.)	400	53.0	20.0	NA	18	445
●★■ Pecan, homemade (⅙ of 9″ pie)	577	70.8	31.6	4.4	87	458
●★■ Pineapple chiffon, homemade (⅙ of 9″ pie)	311	42.2	13.1	3.5	164	414
●★■ Pineapple custard, homemade (⅙ of 9″ pie)	334	48.8	13.2	4.0	84	424
●★ Pineapple, homemade (⅙ of 9″ pie)	400	60.2	16.9	4.2	0	643
●★■ Pumpkin, frozen, *Banquet* (20 oz.)	1236	193.9	41.1	NA	NA	1327
●★■ Pumpkin, frozen, *Morton* (4 oz.)	230	36.0	8.0	NA	44	310
●★■ Pumpkin, homemade (⅙ of 9″ pie)	321	37.2	17.0	6.0	93	487
●★ Raisin, homemade (⅙ of 9″ pie)	427	67.9	16.9	4.2	0	450
●★ Rhubarb, homemade (⅙ of 9″ pie)	400	60.4	16.9	4.2	0	639
●★ Strawberry, homemade (⅙ of 9″ pie)	246	38.3	9.8	2.4	0	360
●★■ Sweetpotato, homemade (⅙ of 9″ pie)	324	36.0	17.2	6.2	82	497
●★ Vanilla marble, mix, *No Bake Desserts, Pillsbury* (⅙ package)	215	42.0	5.0	NA	NA	385

Alerts: ● Sodium ★ Sugar ■ Cholesterol

Poultry

All poultry contains cholesterol and sodium in varying, yet *relatively* substantial, amounts. If you are restricting either of these two food constituents in your diet, you should maintain an awareness of your cholesterol or sodium intake when you consume poultry. We have assigned an alert to a particular item only when the cholesterol or sodium content may be considered unacceptably high—due to the nature of the food or the method or processing or preparation—when compared to other poultry items.

Food Description	Calories	Carbohydrates (grams)	Fat (grams)	Saturated Fat (grams)	Cholesterol (milligrams)	Sodium (milligrams)
Duck, domestic, roasted, meat and skin (6.1 oz.)	583	0	49.1	16.7	145	103
Duck, domestic, roasted, meat only (3½ oz.)	201	0	11.2	4.2	89	65
Goose, roasted, with skin and giblets (8.5 oz.)	1022	0	86.4	26.4	209	297
■ Goose, Pâté de foie gras, canned (1 Tbsp.)	10	0.6	5.7	1.6	57	8
Goose, roasted (3 oz.)	198	0	8.3	2.6	74	105
CHICKEN						
• Breasts, batter dipped, frozen, *Weaver* (3½ oz.)	242	13.1	13.6	NA	NA	NA
• Breasts, Dutch fry, frozen, *Weaver* (3½ oz.)	263	13.7	14.8	NA	NA	NA
• Breast, frozen, *Swanson* (3.2 oz.)	250	8.0	16.0	NA	NA	385
Broiler, broiled (10.4 oz.)	240	0	6.7	6.7	153	116
• Canned (5½ oz. can)	309	0	18.3	5.8	123	695
• Canned, chunks, *Swanson* (2½ oz.)	110	0	6.0	NA	NA	385
• Canned, chunk thigh meat, *Swanson* (2½ oz.)	120	0	7.0	NA	NA	430
• Canned, chunk white, in broth, *Swanson* (2½ oz.)	110	0	5.0	NA	NA	415
Canned, *Featherweight* (5 oz.)	NA	NA	NA	NA	NA	100
Dark meat, roasted, chopped or diced (1 cup)	246	0	8.8	2.8	127	120

Alerts: • Sodium ★ Sugar ■ Cholesterol

Food Description	Calories	Carbohydrates (grams)	Fat (grams)	Saturated Fat (grams)	Cholesterol (milligrams)	Sodium (milligrams)
● Drumsticks, Dutch fry, frozen, *Weaver* (3½ oz.)	217	13.4	10.2	NA	NA	NA
●★ Fried, frozen, *Touch of Honey,* *Weaver* (3½ oz.)	249	13.4	13.0	NA	NA	NA
● Frozen, take-out style, *Swanson* (4 oz.)	260	8.0	16.0	NA	NA	1090
Fryer, fried (1 back)	139	2.7	8.5	2.6	37	35
Fryer, fried (½ breast, ribless)	160	1.2	5.1	1.5	63	53
Fryer, fried (1 drumstick)	88	0.4	3.8	1.1	34	53
Fryer, fried (1 neck)	127	2.0	7.6	2.4	40	38
Fryer, fried (1 rib section)	41	0.8	2.1	0.6	71	9
Fryer, fried (1 thigh)	122	1.3	5.9	1.8	47	45
Fryer, fried (1 wing)	82	0.8	4.5	1.4	28	26
Fryer, fried, dark meat (1.4 oz. piece)	88	0.6	3.7	1.1	36	35
Fryer, fried, light meat (1.8 oz. piece)	99	0.6	3.1	0.9	40	34
■ Fryer, fried, with skin and giblets (8 oz.)	565	6.6	26.8	8.0	368	177
■ Gizzard, simmered (11.8 oz.)	497	2.4	11.1	3.4	655	191
■ Gizzard, simmered, chopped (1 cup)	215	1.0	4.8	1.5	283	82
■ Heart, simmered, diced (1 cup)	251	0.1	10.4	2.9	335	100
Hens and cocks, stewed, dark meat, skinned (1 cup)	290	0	13.3	4.3	127	89
Hens and cocks, stewed, light meat, skinned (1 cup)	252	0	6.6	2.1	111	67
■ Hens and cocks, stewed, with skin and giblets (8 oz.)	708	0	59.5	16.1	306	124
Light meat, roasted, chopped or diced (1 cup)	232	0	4.8	1.5	111	89
■ Liver, fried, chopped (1 cup)	231	4.3	6.2	1.4	1044	85
● Parts, batter dipped, frozen, *Weaver* (3½ oz.)	273	14.4	17.8	NA	NA	NA
● Parts, Dutch fry, frozen, *Weaver* (3½ oz.)	287	16.5	17.5	NA	NA	NA
● Parts, fried, frozen, *Swanson* (3.2 oz.)	260	10.0	17.0	NA	NA	465
● Patty, *Rondelet* (1 patty)	174	11.2	7.5	NA	NA	NA
Roaster, roasted, dark meat, diced (1 cup)	258	0	9.1	2.9	127	123
Roaster, roasted, light meat, diced (1 cup)	255	0	6.9	2.2	111	92
■ Roaster, roasted, with skin and giblets (8.4 oz.)	576	0	33.3	10.7	324	183

Alerts: ● Sodium ★ Sugar ■ Cholesterol

Food Description	Calories	Carbohydrates (grams)	Fat (grams)	Saturated Fat (grams)	Cholesterol (milligrams)	Sodium (milligrams)
• Thighs and drumsticks, batter dipped, frozen, *Weaver* (3½ oz.)	245	12.6	14.4	NA	NA	NA
• Thighs and drumsticks, Dutch fry, frozen, *Weaver* (3½ oz.)	259	15.4	14.5	NA	NA	NA
• Thighs and drumsticks, frozen, *Swanson* (3.2 oz.)	260	7.0	18.0	NA	NA	380
• Wing sections, frozen, *Swanson* (3.2 oz.)	290	12.0	20.0	NA	NA	360
TURKEY						
•★ Breast, boneless, barbecued, *Louis Rich* (2 oz.)	80	1.0	3.0	NA	NA	NA
• Breast, boneless, roasted, *Louis Rich* (2 oz.)	100	0	4.0	NA	NA	NA
Breast, fresh, *Louis Rich* (3 oz.)	120	0	5.0	NA	NA	NA
Breast, fresh, slices, *Louis Rich* (3 oz.)	100	0	1.0	NA	NA	NA
Breast, fresh, tenderloins, *Louis Rich* (3 oz.)	100	0	1.0	NA	NA	NA
Breast, fresh, tenderloin steaks, *Louis Rich* (3 oz.)	100	0	1.0	NA	NA	NA
Breast half, boneless, fresh, *Louis Rich* (3 oz.)	120	0	5.0	NA	NA	NA
Breast half, fresh, with ribs, back and neck skin, *Louis Rich* (3 oz.)	120	0	5.0	NA	NA	NA
• Canned (5½ oz.)	315	0	19.5	5.7	139	140
• Canned, chunks, *Swanson* (2½ oz.)	120	0	7.0	NA	NA	380
Dark meat, roasted (3 oz. piece)	173	0	7.1	2.1	86	84
Dark meat, roasted, diced (1 cup)	284	0	11.6	3.4	141	138
Dark meat, roasted, ground (1 cup)	223	0	9.1	2.7	111	108
Drumstick, fresh, *Louis Rich* (3 oz.)	110	0	4.0	NA	NA	NA
■ Giblets, simmered, diced (1 cup)	338	2.3	22.3	5.8	682	79
■ Gizzard, simmered, chopped (1 cup)	284	1.6	12.5	2.9	332	73
■ Heart, simmered, diced (1 cup)	313	0.3	19.1	5.8	345	88

Alerts: • Sodium ★ Sugar ■ Cholesterol

Food Description	Calories	Carbohydrates (grams)	Fat (grams)	Saturated Fat (grams)	Cholesterol (milligrams)	Sodium (milligrams)
•Hickory smoked, boneless, *Louis Rich* (2 oz.)	75	1.0	4.0	NA	NA	NA
•Hickory smoked, breast, boneless, *Louis Rich* (2 oz.)	80	1	3	NA	NA	NA
•Hickory smoked, drumsticks, *Louis Rich* (2 oz.)	100	0	5.0	NA	NA	NA
•Hickory smoked, wings, *Louis Rich* (2 oz.)	110	0	5.0	NA	NA	NA
Hind quarter, fresh, with leg, thigh, back and tail, *Louis Rich* (3 oz.)	180	0	12.0	NA	NA	NA
Light meat, roasted (3 oz. slice)	150	0	3.3	1.0	65	69
Light meat, roasted, diced (1 cup)	246	0	5.5	1.6	108	114
Light meat, roasted, ground (1 cup)	194	0	4.3	1.2	85	90
■Liver, simmered, chopped (1 cup)	244	4.3	6.7	1.4	839	77
■Roasted (8.6 oz.)	644	0	40.2	11.7	257	215
Roasted (3 oz. slice)	161	0	5.2	1.5	76	110
Thigh, fresh, *Louis Rich* (3 oz.)	170	0	11.0	NA	NA	NA
Wing, fresh, *Drumettes*, *Louis Rich* (3 oz.)	120	0	7.0	NA	NA	NA
Wing, fresh, *Louis Rich* (3 oz.)	130	0	6.0	NA	NA	NA
Wing, fresh, second part, *Louis Rich* (3 oz.)	140	0	9.0	NA	NA	NA
•Young, butter basted, roasted, *Land O' Lakes* (3 oz.)	140	0	8.0	3.0	85	137
Young, roasted, *Land O' Lakes* (3 oz.)	120	0	5.0	2.0	79	45
•Young, self-basting, roasted, *Land O' Lakes* (3 oz.)	120	0	5.0	2.0	77	144

Alerts: • Sodium ★ Sugar ■ Cholesterol

Salad Dressings

Food Description	Calories	Carbohydrates (grams)	Fat (grams)	Saturated Fat (grams)	Cholesterol (milligrams)	Sodium (milligrams)
●★Blue cheese, *Dieter's Gourmet* (1 Tbsp.)	14	2.0	1.0	Tr.	0	NA
●Blue cheese flavor, low calorie, *Featherweight* (1 Tbsp.)	4	1.0	0	0	NA	NA
●Blue cheese, mix, *Good Seasons* (1 Tbsp.)	4	0	0	0	NA	211
●Blue cheese, mix, *Thick 'N Creamy, Good Seasons* (1 Tbsp.)	12	0	1.0	NA	NA	80
●★Blue cheese, *Wish-Bone Lite* (1 Tbsp.)	40	3.0	3.0	NA	0	NA
★Blue cheese, commercial, with no salt (1 Tbsp.)	76	1.1	7.8	1.6	3	5
●★Blue cheese, commercial, with salt (1 Tbsp.)	76	1.1	7.8	1.6	3	164
●★*Buttermilk Farm Style,* mix, *Good Seasons* (1 Tbsp.)	4	1.0	0	0	NA	90
●★Caesar, low calorie, *Pfeiffer* (1 oz.)	20	2.0	1.0	NA	NA	NA
●★Caesar, *Seven Seas* (1 Tbsp.)	60	1.0	7.0	1.0	0	260
●★Caesar, *Wish-Bone* (1 Tbsp.)	80	1.0	8.0	NA	0	NA
●★*California onion, Wish-Bone* (1 Tbsp.)	70	1.0	8.0	NA	0	NA
●★*Capri, Seven Seas* (1 Tbsp.)	70	3.0	6.0	1.0	0	130
●★*Cheese garlic,* mix, *Good Seasons* (1 Tbsp.)	4	0	0	0	NA	166
●★*Cheese Italian,* mix, *Good Seasons* (1 Tbsp.)	6	1.0	0	0	NA	180
●★Chef style, reduced calorie, *Kraft* (1 Tbsp.)	18	3.0	1.0	0	0	115
●★*Chunky Blue Cheese, Wish-Bone* (1 Tbsp.)	70	1.0	7.0	NA	0	NA
●★Creamy bacon, *Seven Seas* (1 Tbsp.)	60	1.0	6.0	1.0	0	205
●★*Creamy Cucumber and Onion, Featherweight* (1 Tbsp.)	4	1.0	0	0	0	NA

Alerts: ● Sodium ★ Sugar ■ Cholesterol

Food Description	Calories	Carbohydrates (grams)	Fat (grams)	Saturated Fat (grams)	Cholesterol (milligrams)	Sodium (milligrams)
●★■ Creamy cucumber, reduced calorie, *Kraft* (1 Tbsp.)	30	1.0	3.0	1.0	30	230
●★ Creamy cucumber, *Wish-Bone* (1 Tbsp.)	80	2.0	8.0	NA	0	NA
●★ Creamy cucumber, *Wish-Bone Lite* (1 Tbsp.)	40	1.0	4.0	NA	0	NA
●★ Creamy French, *Seven Seas* (1 Tbsp.)	60	2.0	6.0	1.0	0	265
●★ Creamy garlic, *Wish-Bone* (1 Tbsp.)	80	2.0	8.0	NA	0	NA
●★ Creamy Italian, *Seven Seas* (1 Tbsp.)	70	1.0	7.0	1.0	0	255
●★ Creamy Italian, *Wish-Bone* (1 Tbsp.)	80	2.0	8.0	NA	NA	NA
●★ Creamy Italian, *Wish-Bone Lite* (1 Tbsp.)	30	1.0	3.0	NA	0	NA
●★ *Creamy Onion 'N Chive, Seven Seas* (1 Tbsp.)	60	1.0	7.0	1.0	0	190
●★ Creamy Russian, low calorie, *Featherweight* (1 Tbsp.)	6	1.0	0	0	NA	NA
●★ Creamy Russian, *Seven Seas* (1 Tbsp.)	80	1.0	8.0	1.0	0	115
●★ Deluxe French, *Wish-Bone* (1 Tbsp.)	60	3.0	5.0	NA	0	NA
●★ *Family Style French, Seven Seas* (1 Tbsp.)	10	3.0	6.0	1.0	0	135
● *Family Style Italian, Seven Seas* (1 Tbsp.)	70	0	7.0	1.0	0	170
● *Farm Style, mix, Good Seasons* (1 oz.)	2	0	0	0	0	155
● French, homemade, with corn oil (1 Tbsp.)	88	0.5	9.8	1.0	0	92
French, imitation, low sodium, *Featherweight* (1 Tbsp.)	60	0	6.0	NA	0	4
●★ French, low calorie, *Pfeiffer* (1 oz.)	35	5.0	2.0	NA	NA	NA
★ French, commercial, low fat, with no salt (1 Tbsp.)	15	2.5	0.7	0.1	0	5
●★ French, commercial, low fat, with salt (1 Tbsp.)	15	2.5	0.7	0.1	0	125
●★ *French, mix, Good Seasons* (1 Tbsp.)	14	3.0	0	0	NA	203
●★ *French, mix, Thick 'N Creamy, Good Seasons* (1 Tbsp.)	16	3.0	0	0	0	262
●★ French style, *Dieter's Gourmet* (½ oz. packet)	14	2.0	1.0	Tr.	0	NA

Alerts: ● Sodium ★ Sugar ■ Cholesterol

Food Description	Calories	Carbohydrates (grams)	Fat (grams)	Saturated Fat (grams)	Cholesterol (milligrams)	Sodium (milligrams)
●★French style, low calorie, *Featherweight* (1 Tbsp.)	1	1.0	0	0	0	NA
●★French style, *Weight Watchers* (¼ cup)	10	1.0	0	NA	NA	NA
●★French style, *Wish-Bone Lite* (1 Tbsp.)	30	2.0	2.0	NA	0	NA
★French, commercial, with no salt (1 Tbsp.)	66	2.8	6.2	1.1	0	5
●★French, commercial, with salt (1 Tbsp.)	66	2.8	6.2	1.1	0	219
●★Garlic, *Dieter's Gourmet* (1 Tbsp.)	14	2.0	1.0	Tr.	0	NA
●★Garlic French, *Wish-Bone* (1 Tbsp.)	60	2.0	6.0	NA	0	NA
● Garlic, mix, *Good Seasons* (1 Tbsp.)	2	0	0	0	0	221
●★Green goddess, *Seven Seas* (1 Tbsp.)	60	0	7.0	1.0	0	140
●★Green goddess, *Wish-Bone* (1 Tbsp.)	70	1.0	7.0	NA	0	NA
●★Herb, *Dieter's Gourmet* (1 Tbsp.)	14	2.0	1.0	Tr.	0	NA
●★Herbs and spices, *Seven Seas* (1 Tbsp.)	60	1.0	6.0	1.0	0	160
Italian						
★Commercial, with no salt (1 Tbsp.)	83	1.0	9.0	1.6	0	5
●★Commercial, with salt (1 Tbsp.)	83	1.0	9.0	1.6	0	313
●★Low calorie, *Featherweight* (1 Tbsp.)	4	1.0	0	0	0	NA
●★Low calorie, mix, *Good Seasons* (1 Tbsp.)	7	2.0	0	0	0	148
●★Low calorie, *Pfeiffer* (1 oz.)	20	3.0	1.0	NA	NA	NA
★Low calorie, commercial, with no salt (1 Tbsp.)	8	0.4	0.7	0.1	0	5
●★Low calorie, commercial, with salt (1 Tbsp.)	8	0.4	0.7	0.1	0	118
●★Mix, *Good Seasons* (1 Tbsp.)	4	1.0	0	0	0	200
●★Mix, *Thick 'N Creamy, Good Seasons* (1 Tbsp.)	10	1.0	0	0	0	231
●★*Weight Watchers* (1 Tbsp.)	50	2.0	5.0	1.0	5	124
●★*Wish-Bone* (1 Tbsp.)	80	1.0	8.0	NA	0	NA
●★*Wish-Bone Lite* (1 Tbsp.)	30	1.0	3.0	NA	0	NA
●★■ Mayonnaise (1 Tbsp.)	101	0.3	11.2	2.0	10	83

Alerts: ● Sodium ★ Sugar ■ Cholesterol

Food Description	Calories	Carbohydrates (grams)	Fat (grams)	Saturated Fat (grams)	Cholesterol (milligrams)	Sodium (milligrams)
★■ Mayonnaise base, low fat (1 Tbsp.)	22	0.8	2.0	0.4	8	18
●★■ Mayonnaise base, with salt (1 Tbsp.)	65	2.2	6.3	1.2	8	87
●★■ Mayonnaise, *Hellman's* (1 Tbsp.)	100	0	11.0	2.0	10	80
Mayonnaise, imitation, *Featherweight* (1 Tbsp.)	100	0	11.0	NA	NA	3
●★ Mayonnaise, imitation, *Spred Lite, Batter-Lite* (1 Tbsp.)	44	1.0	4.0	NA	NA	46
●★■ Mayonnaise, *Kraft* (1 Tbsp.)	100	0	4.0	2.0	5	70
●★■ Mayonnaise, reduced calorie, *Weight Watchers* (1 Tbsp.)	40	1.0	4.0	1.0	5	109
★■ Mayonnaise, with no salt (1 Tbsp.)	101	0.3	11.2	2.0	10	4
●★ Mild Italian, mix, *Good Seasons* (1 Tbsp.)	6	1.0	0	0	0	148
●★■ *Miracle Whip* (1 Tbsp.)	70	2.0	0.7	1.0	5	90
● *Old Fashion French,* mix, *Good Seaons* (1 Tbsp.)	2	0	0	0	0	255
●★ Onion, mix, *Good Seasons* (1 Tbsp.)	4	1.0	0	0	0	142
●★ Red wine, low calorie, *Pfeiffer* (1 oz.)	20	2.0	1.0	NA	NA	NA
●★ Red wine, vinegar and oil, *Seven Seas* (1 Tbsp.)	60	1.0	7.0	1.0	0	265
●★ Red wine vinegar, low calorie, *Featherweight* (1 Tbsp.)	6	1.0	0	0	0	NA
●★ *Riviera French,* mix, *Good Seasons* (1 Tbsp.)	10	2.0	0	0	0	278
★ Roquefort cheese, commercial, with no salt (1 Tbsp.)	76	1.1	7.8	1.6	3	5
●★ Roquefort cheese, commercial, with salt (1 Tbsp.)	76	1.1	7.8	1.6	3	164
●★ Russian, low calorie, *Pfeiffer* (1 oz.)	30	4.0	1.0	NA	NA	NA
●★■ Russian, *Weight Watchers* (1 Tbsp.)	50	2.0	5.0	1.0	5	114
●★ Russian, *Wish-Bone* (1 Tbsp.)	50	7.0	2.0	NA	0	NA
●★ Russian, *Wish-Bone Lite* (1 Tbsp.)	25	5.0	1.0	NA	0	NA
★■ Russian, commercial, with no salt (1 Tbsp.)	74	1.6	7.6	1.4	8	5

Alerts: ● Sodium ★ Sugar ■ Cholesterol

Food Description	Calories	Carbohydrates (grams)	Fat (grams)	Saturated Fat (grams)	Cholesterol (milligrams)	Sodium (milligrams)
●★■ Russian, commercial, with salt (1 Tbsp.)	74	1.6	7.6	1.4	8	130
●★■ *Spin Blend, Hellman's* (1 Tbsp.)	60	3.0	5.0	1.0	10	110
●★ *Sweet 'N Spicy French, Wish-Bone* (1 Tbsp.)	60	3.0	5.0	NA	0	NA
●★ *Sweet 'N Spicy French, Wish-Bone Lite* (1 Tbsp.)	30	4.0	2.0	NA	0	NA
Thousand Island						
★■ Commercial, with no salt (1 Tbsp.)	80	2.5	8.0	1.4	8	5
●★■ Commercial, with salt (1 Tbsp.)	80	2.5	8.0	1.4	8	112
●★ *Dieter's Gourmet* (1 Tbsp.)	14	2.0	1.0	Tr.	0	NA
●★■ Low calorie, *Pfeiffer* (1 oz.)	30	4.0	1.0	NA	NA	NA
★■ Low fat, commercial, with no salt (1 Tbsp.)	27	2.3	2.1	0.4	8	5
●★■ Low fat, commercial, with salt (1 Tbsp.)	27	2.3	2.1	0.4	8	105
★ Mix, *Thick 'N Creamy, Good Seasons* (1 Tbsp.)	4	1.0	0	0	0	0
●★■ *Seven Seas* (1 Tbsp.)	50	2.0	5.0	1.0	320	350
●★■ *Weight Watchers* (1 Tbsp.)	50	2.0	5.0	1.0	5	114
●★■ *Wish-Bone* (1 Tbsp.)	70	3.0	6.0	NA	5	NA
●★■ *Wish-Bone Lite* (1 Tbsp.)	25	3.0	2.0	NA	5	NA
2 Calorie Low Sodium, Featherweight (1 Tbsp.)	2	0	0	0	0	6
●★ Vinaigrette, *Dieter's Gourmet* (1 Tbsp.)	14	2.0	1.0	Tr.	0	NA
●★ *Viva Bell Pepper, Seven Seas* (1 Tbsp.)	45	1.0	5.0	1.0	0	180
●★ *Viva Caesar, Seven Seas* (1 Tbsp.)	60	1.0	6.0	1.0	0	205
●★ *Viva Italian, Seven Seas* (1 Tbsp.)	70	1.0	7.0	1.0	0	400
●★ Yogurt blue cheese, reduced calorie, *Henri's* (1 Tbsp.)	30	4.0	2.0	NA	NA	NA
●★ Yogurt cucumber and onion, reduced calorie, *Henri's* (1 Tbsp.)	35	5.0	2.0	NA	NA	NA
●★ Yogurt French style, reduced calorie, *Henri's* (1 Tbsp.)	40	6.0	2.0	NA	NA	NA
●★ Yogurt garlic, reduced calorie, *Henri's* (1 Tbsp.)	35	5.0	2.0	NA	NA	NA

Alerts: ● Sodium ★ Sugar ■ Cholesterol

Food Description	Calories	Carbohydrates (grams)	Fat (grams)	Saturated Fat (grams)	Cholesterol (milligrams)	Sodium (milligrams)
●★■ Yogurt Thousand Island, reduced calorie, *Henri's* (1 Tbsp.)	30	4.0	2.0	NA	NA	NA

Sausages and Luncheon Meats

All meats, including sausages and luncheon meats, contain cholesterol and sodium in varying, yet *relatively* substantial, amounts. If you are restricting either of these two food constituents in your diet, you should maintain an awareness of your cholesterol or sodium intake when you consume these foods. We have assigned an alert to a particular item only when the cholesterol or sodium content may be considered unacceptably high—due to the nature of the food or the method of processing—when compared to other meats.

Food Description	Calories	Carbohydrates (grams)	Fat (grams)	Saturated Fat (grams)	Cholesterol (milligrams)	Sodium (milligrams)
● Baked-ham loaf, 95% fat free, smoked, *Oscar Mayer* (1 slice)	25	0	1.0	0.3	13	295
●★ Bar-B-Q Loaf, 90% fat free, *Oscar Mayer* (1 oz. slice)	45	1.7	2.8	1.0	11	369
● Beef, dried, sliced, canned, *Armour* (1¼ oz.)	60	1.0	1.0	NA	NA	1520
● Beef, *Eckrich Slender Sliced* (1.5 oz.)	60	1.0	3.0	NA	NA	NA
● Beef loaf, smoked, *Carl Buddig* (1 oz.)	40	0	2.0	0.4	16	356
● Beer salami, beef, *Oscar Mayer* (0.8 oz. slice)	75	0.2	7.1	3.3	14	234
● Beer salami, *Oscar Mayer* (0.8 oz. slice)	55	0.4	4.4	1.5	13	282
● Berliner sausage (1 oz.)	65	0.7	4.9	1.7	13	368
Blood sausage (1 oz.)	112	0.1	10.5	4.0	17	18
Blood sausage (1 slice)	32	0	3.0	1.1	5	5
● Bockwurst (link)	172	0.4	15.4	6.5	42	715
● Bockwurst (1 lb.)	1198	2.7	107.5	45.4	295	4989
● Bologna (1 oz.)	86	0.3	7.8	3.1	18	368
● Bologna-and-cheese, *Oscar Mayer* (0.8 oz. slice)	75	0.6	6.7	2.7	14	247
● Bologna, beef, *Oscar Mayer* (0.8 oz. slice)	75	0.6	6.7	2.9	13	239

Alerts: ● Sodium ★ Sugar ■ Cholesterol

Food Description	Calories	Carbohydrates (grams)	Fat (grams)	Saturated Fat (grams)	Cholesterol (milligrams)	Sodium (milligrams)
• Bologna, beef, lower fat, *Best's Kosher* (1½ oz.)	100	2.0	8.0	NA	NA	978
• Bologna, beef, smoke flavored, *Eckrich* (2 slices)	190	3.0	16.0	NA	NA	NA
• Bologna, *Eckrich* (2 oz.)	190	3.0	17.0	NA	NA	NA
• Bologna, garlic, *Eckrich* (2 oz.)	190	3.0	17.0	NA	NA	NA
• Bologna, regular, *Oscar Mayer* (0.8 oz. slice)	75	0.4	6.9	2.8	13	241
• Bologna, ring, pickled, *Eckrich* (2 oz.)	190	3.0	17.0	NA	NA	NA
• Bologna, with no binders, (1 oz. slice)	79	1.0	6.5	2.8	18	368
• Bratwurst, cooked (3 oz. link)	256	1.8	22.0	7.9	51	473
•■ Braunschweiger (1 oz. slice)	90	0.7	7.8	2.8	45	368
• Brown-and-serve sausage, frozen (1 oz. patty)	111	0.8	10.2	3.7	18	271
• Brown-and-serve sausage, frozen (¾ oz. link)	83	0.6	7.6	2.7	13	201
• Canadian bacon, 93% fat free, *Oscar Mayer* (1 oz. slice)	40	0	2.0	0.6	12	393
• Cervelat (5⅓ oz.)	677	2.5	56.4	24.0	98	1650
• Chipped beef, uncooked (1 oz.)	58	0	1.8	0.9	18	1219
• Chicken bologna, *Longacre Family* (2 slices)	130	0	11.0	NA	NA	NA
• Chicken bologna, *Weaver* (3½ oz.)	256	3.5	21.4	NA	NA	NA
• Chicken, *Eckrich Slender Sliced* (1.5 oz.)	70	2.0	4.0	NA	NA	NA
•■ Chicken-liver pâté, canned (1 Tbsp.)	26	0.9	1.7	NA	NA	NA
• Chicken loaf, smoked, sliced, *Carl Buddig* (1 oz.)	45	0	3.0	0.8	12	255
• Chicken roll, light meat (2 oz.)	90	1.4	4.2	1.2	28	331
• Chicken roll, *Weaver* (3½ oz.)	141	2.1	6.3	NA	NA	NA
• Chicken roll, white meat, *Longacre Family* (2 slices)	84	0.2	6.0	NA	NA	NA
• Chicken spread, canned (1 oz.)	55	1.5	3.3	NA	NA	NA
• Chopped beef, canned, *Armour* (3 oz.)	290	3.0	26.0	NA	NA	1068
• Chopped ham, canned, *Armour* (3 oz.)	180	3.0	12.0	NA	NA	1148
• Chopped-ham loaf, *Oscar Mayer* (1 oz. slice)	65	0.8	4.5	1.6	14	373

Alerts: • Sodium ★ Sugar ■ Cholesterol

Food Description	Calories	Carbohydrates (grams)	Fat (grams)	Saturated Fat (grams)	Cholesterol (milligrams)	Sodium (milligrams)
• Chopped-ham loaf, smoke flavored, *Eckrich* (2 slices)	100	1.0	5.0	NA	NA	NA
• Corned beef, *Eckrich Slender Sliced* (1.5 oz.)	60	2.0	3.0	NA	NA	NA
• Corned beef, smoked, sliced, *Carl Buddig* (1 oz.)	40	0	2.0	0.4	16	305
• Cotto salami, beef, *Oscar Mayer* (1 oz. slice)	50	0.6	3.9	1.7	14	279
• Cotto salami, regular, *Oscar Mayer* (1 oz. slice)	50	0.4	4.1	1.7	14	245
• Country-style sausage (1 lb.)	1565	0	141.1	50.8	281	4345
• Deviled ham, canned (4½ oz.)	449	0	41.3	14.9	83	1579
• Gourmet loaf, *Eckrich* (2 oz.)	70	4.0	2.0	NA	NA	NA
• Ham-and-cheese loaf, *Eckrich* (2 oz.)	140	2.0	11.0	NA	NA	NA
• Ham-and-cheese loaf, *Oscar Mayer* (1 oz. slice)	75	0.6	4.5	2.4	16	365
• Ham-and-cheese spread (1 Tbsp.)	37	0.3	2.8	1.3	9	179
• Ham, boiled, luncheon meat (1 oz.)	66	0	4.8	1.7	25	349
• Ham, boneless, smoked, *Oscar Mayer Jubilee* (1 oz.)	50	0.2	3.1	1.2	16	386
• Ham, cooked, *Eckrich* (1 slice)	40	1.0	1.0	NA	NA	NA
• Ham, formed, canned, *Oscar Mayer Jubilee* (1 oz.)	30	0.1	1.1	0.4	11	341
• Ham loaf, *Eckrich* (2 oz.)	160	1.0	13.0	NA	NA	NA
• Ham loaf, smoked, sliced, *Carl Buddig* (1 oz.)	45	0	3.0	1.3	20	377
• Ham roll sausage, 92% fat free, *Oscar Mayer* (0.8 oz. slice)	35	0.5	1.8	0.7	11	270
• Ham-salad spread (1 Tbsp.)	32	1.6	2.3	0.8	6	137
• Ham, slice or steak, smoked, formed, *Oscar Mayer Jubilee* (1 oz.)	30	0	1.1	0.4	14	373
• Ham steak, 95% fat free, *Oscar Mayer* (2 oz. slice)	70	0	2.8	0.9	26	741
• Head cheese (8 oz.)	608	2.3	49.9	18.0	148	2497
• Head cheese, *Oscar Mayer* (1 oz. slice)	55	0	3.9	1.3	25	352
Hot Dogs						
• Hot dog (2 oz. frank)	176	1.0	15.7	6.8	37	627
• Hot dog, *Eckrich* (1.2 oz. frank)	120	2.0	11.0	NA	NA	NA
• Beef (2 oz. frank)	184	1.4	16.8	6.8	27	584

Alerts: • Sodium ★ Sugar ■ Cholesterol

Food Description	Calories	Carbohydrates (grams)	Fat (grams)	Saturated Fat (grams)	Cholesterol (milligrams)	Sodium (milligrams)
• Beef, *Eckrich* (1.2 oz. frank)	120	3.0	13.0	NA	NA	NA
• Beef, *Eckrich* (1 jumbo frank)	190	3.0	17.0	NA	NA	NA
• Beef flavor, lower fat, *Best's Kosher* (1 link)	110	2.0	8.0	NA	NA	NA
• Beef, *Oscar Mayer* (1 frank)	145	0.8	13.5	5.2	24	514
• Canned, drained (12 oz. net)	751	0.7	61.5	27.2	211	3740
• Chicken (1.6 oz. frank)	116	3.1	8.8	2.5	45	617
• Chicken, lower fat, *Holly Farms* (1 frank)	150	2.0	13.0	NA	NA	NA
• Chicken, lower fat, *Longacre Family* (2 oz.)	120	0	10.0	NA	60	NA
• Chicken, lower fat, *Weaver* (1 frank)	120	2.0	11.0	NA	65	650
• Corn, heated, *Oscar Mayer* (1 frank)	330	27.3	20.0	8.4	37	1252
• Turkey (1.6 oz. frank)	102	0.7	8.0	NA	48	642
• Turkey, *Louis Rich* (1 large frank)	130	2.0	11.0	NA	NA	NA
• Turkey, lower fat, *Longacre Family* (1.6 oz. frank)	110	0	10.0	NA	25	NA
• With nonfat dry milk added (1 medium frank)	135	1.5	11.5	5.0	29	495
• With no binders, smoked (1 medium frank)	101	0.9	8.7	3.7	22	374
• With cheese, *Oscar Mayer* (1 frank)	145	0.7	13.5	5.3	31	551
• Honey loaf (2 oz.)	73	3.0	2.5	0.8	19	749
• Honey loaf, 95% fat free, *Oscar Mayer* (1 oz. slice)	35	1.4	1.1	0.4	10	373
• Honey roll sausage, beef, 90% fat free, *Oscar Mayer* (0.8 oz. slice)	40	0.7	2.3	1.0	12	304
• Honey-style loaf, *Eckrich* (2 slices)	90	4	4	NA	NA	NA
• Italian sausage, cooked (3 oz. link)	268	1.2	21.3	7.5	65	765
• Knockwurst (1 link)	189	1.5	15.8	6.8	44	748
• Knockwurst (12 oz.)	945	7.5	78.9	34.0	221	3740
•■ Liver cheese, pork fat wrapped, *Oscar Mayer* (1⅓ oz. slice)	115	0.6	9.9	3.6	69	456
•■ Liver sausage, *Oscar Mayer* (1 oz.)	95	0.8	8.7	3.1	39	330
•■ Liverwurst (8 oz.)	697	4.1	58.1	20.4	362	2495

Alerts: • Sodium ★ Sugar ■ Cholesterol

Food Description	Calories	Carbohydrates (grams)	Fat (grams)	Saturated Fat (grams)	Cholesterol (milligrams)	Sodium (milligrams)
●Luncheon meat, *Oscar Mayer* (1 oz. slice)	95	0.4	9.0	3.3	16	358
●Luncheon sausage, pork-and-beef (1 oz.)	74	0.5	5.9	2.2	18	335
●Luxury loaf, 95% fat free, *Oscar Mayer* (1 oz. slice)	40	1.5	1.4	0.5	11	328
●Meat-loaf luncheon meat (8 oz.)	454	7.5	30.0	13.6	148	2948
●Meat, potted (3 oz.)	223	0	17.3	8.1	70	1170
●Meat, potted (1 Tbsp.)	32	0	2.5	1.2	10	169
●Minced ham, luncheon meat (8 oz.)	517	10.0	38.4	13.8	202	2948
●Mortadella (8 oz.)	715	1.4	56.7	22.7	148	2948
●New England sausage, 92% fat free, *Oscar Mayer* (0.8 oz.)	35	0.6	1.8	0.6	14	295
●Old fashioned loaf, *Eckrich* (2 slices)	150	4.0	12.0	NA	NA	NA
●Old fashioned loaf, *Oscar Mayer* (1 oz. slice)	15	2.3	4.2	1.5	13	343
●Olive loaf (1 oz. slice)	67	2.6	4.7	1.7	11	421
●Olive loaf, *Eckrich* (2 oz.)	170	3.0	15.0	NA	NA	NA
●Olive loaf, *Oscar Mayer* (1 oz. slice)	65	2.7	4.5	1.7	11	400
●Pastrami, *Eckrich Slender Sliced* (1.5 oz.)	70	2.0	3.0	NA	NA	NA
●Pastrami loaf, smoked, sliced, *Carl Buddig* (1 oz.)	40	0	2.0	0.4	16	354
●Peppered loaf, *Eckrich* (2 oz.)	80	2.0	3.0	NA	NA	NA
●Peppered loaf, 93% fat free, *Oscar Mayer* (1 oz. slice)	40	1.3	2.0	0.7	14	399
●Pepperoni (0.2 oz. slice)	27	0.2	2.4	0.9	NA	112
●Pickle-and-pimiento loaf (1 oz. slice)	74	1.7	6.0	2.2	10	394
●Pickle-and-pimiento loaf, *Oscar Mayer* (1 oz. slice)	65	3.0	4.2	1.7	11	382
●Pickle loaf, *Eckrich* (2 oz.)	170	3.0	15.0	NA	NA	NA
●Picnic loaf, *Oscar Mayer* (1 oz. slice)	65	1.5	4.5	1.7	11	320
●Polish sausage (1 large)	690	2.7	58.6	20.4	141	2951
●Polish sausage (1 small)	231	0.9	19.6	6.8	47	988
●Polish sausage (10″ sausage)	739	3.7	65.2	23.4	158	1989
●Polska kielbasa, *Eckrich* (2 oz.)	200	1.0	19.0	NA	NA	NA
●Pork sausage, canned (8 oz.)	942	5.4	87.2	31.4	152	2174
●Pork sausage, cooked (7.5 oz./yield of 1 lb. raw)	1014	0	94.1	33.9	190	2040

Alerts: ● Sodium ★ Sugar ■ Cholesterol

Food Description	Calories	Carbohydrates (grams)	Fat (grams)	Saturated Fat (grams)	Cholesterol (milligrams)	Sodium (milligrams)
• Pork sausage, cooked, *Oscar Mayer Little Friers* (0.7 oz. link)	80	0.2	7.6	2.6	18	223
• Pork sausage link, cooked (0.5 oz./yield of 1 oz. raw)	62	0	5.7	2.1	12	124
• Pork sausage patty, cooked (1 oz./yield of 2 oz. raw)	129	0	11.9	4.3	24	258
• Pork sausage, *Oscar Mayer Smokie Links* (1½ oz. link)	135	0.6	12.5	4.7	26	396
• Pork sausage, Southern style, cooked, *Oscar Mayer* (1 oz. patty)	125	0	11.3	4.0	27	282
• Salami, beef, lower fat, *Best's Kosher* (1½ oz.)	100	2.0	7.0	NA	NA	978
• Salami, dry (⅛″ slice)	23	0.1	1.9	0.8	3	61
• Salami, dry (8 oz.)	1021	2.7	86.4	36.3	148	2799
• Salami, hard, *Oscar Mayer* (⅓ oz. slice)	35	0.2	2.8	1.0	7	167
• Sandwich spread, canned, *Oscar Mayer* (1 oz.)	65	3.2	5.0	1.8	10	275
• Sausage, *Beef Smokies, Oscar Mayer* (1½ oz. link)	130	0.9	11.6	5.2	30	455
• Sausage, *Cheese Smokies, Oscar Mayer* (1½ oz. link)	140	0.4	12.9	5.1	30	450
• Scrapple (1 slice)	54	3.7	3.4	1.3	11	239
• Scrapple (8 oz.)	488	33.1	30.9	11.4	100	2173
• Smoked ham, *Eckrich Slender Sliced* (1.5 oz.)	80	1.0	4.0	NA	NA	NA
• Smoked pork, *Eckrich Slender Sliced* (1.5 oz.)	70	1.0	3.0	NA	NA	NA
• Smoked sausage, *Eckrich* (2 oz.)	190	1.0	17.0	NA	NA	NA
• Smoked sausage, beef, *Eckrich* (2 oz.)	190	1.0	17.0	NA	NA	NA
• Smoked sausage, skinless, *Eckrich* (2 oz.)	190	2.0	17.0	NA	NA	NA
• Smoked turkey, breast, *Longacre Family* (2 slices)	45	1.0	Tr.	NA	10	201
• *Smok-Y-Links,* beef, *Eckrich* (1.7 oz.)	150	2.0	12.0	NA	NA	NA
• *Smok-Y-Links,* maple flavored, *Eckrich* (1.7 oz.)	150	2.0	13.0	NA	NA	NA
• Spiced ham, chopped, canned (1 slice)	176	0.8	14.9	5.4	53	740
• Spiced ham, chopped, canned (12 oz.)	1000	4.4	84.7	30.5	303	4195

Alerts: • Sodium ★ Sugar ■ Cholesterol

Food Description	Calories	Carbohydrates (grams)	Fat (grams)	Saturated Fat (grams)	Cholesterol (milligrams)	Sodium (milligrams)
• Summer sausage (1 medium slice)	68	0.4	5.4	2.2	14	286
• Summer sausage (8 oz.)	697	3.6	55.6	22.7	148	2951
• Summer sausage, beef, *Oscar Mayer* (0.8 oz. slice)	70	0.7	6.2	2.8	17	317
• Summer sausage, regular, *Oscar Mayer* (0.8 oz. slice)	75	0.2	6.7	2.8	17	340
• Turkey bologna (2 oz.)	113	0.6	8.6	NA	56	498
• Turkey bologna (no pork or beef), *Louis Rich* (2 slices)	140	1.0	12.0	NA	NA	NA
• Turkey breast meat, *Louis Rich* (2 slices)	70	0	2.0	NA	NA	NA
• Turkey breast meat, 98% fat free, *Oscar Mayer* (¾ oz. slice)	20	0	0.4	0.1	8	295
• Turkey breast meat, smoked, *Louis Rich* (2 oz.)	45	1.0	1.0	NA	NA	NA
Turkey breast, unsalted, *Weaver Chef's Gourmet* (3½ oz.)	189	0.6	10.5	NA	NA	NA
• Turkey ham meat, baked, (cured turkey thigh), *Longacre Family* (2 slices)	60	0	3.0	NA	NA	NA
• Turkey ham, smoked, sliced, *Carl Buddig* (1 oz.)	45	0	3.0	0.6	5	418
• Turkey ham, smoked thigh meat (2 oz.)	73	0.2	2.9	1.0	Tr.	565
• Turkey ham (thigh meat), boneless, hickory smoked, *Louis Rich* (2 oz.)	80	1.0	3.0	NA	NA	NA
• Turkey ham, *Weaver* (3½ oz.)	122	0.8	4.5	NA	NA	NA
• Turkey loaf, breast meat (1.5 oz.)	47	0	0.7	0.2	17	608
• Turkey loaf, smoked, sliced, *Carl Buddig* (1 oz.)	45	0	3.0	0.4	5	266
• Turkey luncheon meat, smoked, *Louis Rich* (2 oz.)	90	1.0	4.0	NA	NA	NA
• Turkey pastrami (2 oz.)	80	0.9	3.5	1.0	Tr.	593
• Turkey pastrami, hickory smoked, *Louis Rich* (2 oz.)	70	0	3.0	NA	NA	NA
• Turkey pastrami, *Longacre Family* (2 slices)	60	0	2.0	NA	NA	NA
• Turkey pastrami, *Louis Rich* (2 oz.)	70	0	3.0	NA	NA	NA
• Turkey roll, light meat (1 oz. slice)	42	0.2	2.1	0.6	12	139

Alerts: • Sodium ★ Sugar ■ Cholesterol

Food Description	Calories	Carbohydrates (grams)	Fat (grams)	Saturated Fat (grams)	Cholesterol (milligrams)	Sodium (milligrams)
• Turkey roll, light and dark meat (1 oz. slice)	42	0.6	2.0	0.6	16	166
• Turkey salami (2 oz.)	111	0.3	7.8	NA	46	569
• Turkey salami, *Longacre Family* (2 slices)	70	2.0	4.0	NA	NA	NA
• Turkey salami (no pork or beef), *Louis Rich* (2 slices)	110	1.0	9.0	NA	NA	NA
• Turkey summer sausage, *Louis Rich* (2 oz.)	110	0	8.0	NA	NA	NA
• Vienna sausage, canned, drained (1 sausage)	38	0	3.2	1.1	11	176

Snack Foods

	Calories	Carbohydrates (grams)	Fat (grams)	Saturated Fat (grams)	Cholesterol (milligrams)	Sodium (milligrams)
•★■*Banana Susy Q's, Hostess* (1 cake)	240	38.0	9.0	NA	21	195
•★*Big Wheels, Hostess* (1 cake)	170	21.0	10.0	NA	6	95
• Breadsticks, no salt coating (10 8″ sticks)	192	37.6	1.4	0.3	2	350
• Breadsticks, salt coated (10 8″ sticks)	192	37.6	1.4	0.3	2	837
• Breadsticks, Vienna style (1 6½″ fat stick)	106	20.3	1.1	0.2	1	547
•★ Breakfast bar, almond crunch, *Carnation* (1.51 oz.)	210	20.0	12.0	NA	NA	175
•★ Breakfast bar, butter crunch, *Carnation* (1 bar)	180	19.0	9.0	NA	NA	154
•★ Breakfast bar, caramel nut crunch, *Carnation* (1.35 oz.)	200	19.0	11.0	NA	NA	184
•★ Breakfast bar, chocolate chip, *Carnation* (1 bar)	200	20.0	11.0	NA	NA	163
•★ Breakfast bar, chocolate crunch, *Carnation* (1 bar)	190	18.0	10.0	NA	NA	129
•★ Breakfast bar, malted milk crunch, *Carnation* (1.34 oz.)	190	20.0	10.0	NA	NA	187
•★ Breakfast squares, variety pack, *General Mills* (2 bars)	380	45.0	17.0	Tr.	0	510
•★ Brownie nut bar, *Pepperidge Farm* (1 bar)	190	31.0	7.0	NA	NA	69

Alerts: • Sodium ★ Sugar ■ Cholesterol

Food Description	Calories	Carbohydrates (grams)	Fat (grams)	Saturated Fat (grams)	Cholesterol (milligrams)	Sodium (milligrams)
● *Bugles, General Mills* (1 oz.)	150	18.0	8.0	NA	0	335
●★■ Caramel nut bar, *Figurines* (2 bars)	275	21.0	16.0	NA	NA	210
●★ Cheddar chips, *Lipton Flavor Tree* (1 oz.)	160	12.0	11.0	NA	NA	NA
● Cheese straws, made with vegetable shortening (10 5″ straws)	272	20.7	17.9	6.4	19	432
● *Cheez Curls, Planters* (1 oz.)	160	15.0	10.0	1.0	0	300
★ Cherry yogurt granola bar, *Crunchola* (1 bar)	120	15.0	6.0	4.5	0	32
●★■ *Choco-Dile, Hostess* (1 cake)	250	37.0	11.0	NA	22	225
●★ Chocolate bar, *Carnation Slender* (2 bars)	275	23.0	16.0	NA	NA	358
●★■ Chocolate bar, *Figurines* (2 bars)	275	21.0	16.0	NA	NA	155
●★■ Chocolate caramel bar, *Figurines* (2 bars)	275	21.0	16.0	NA	NA	150
●★ Chocolate caramel nut bar, *Carnation Slender* (2 bars)	275	26.0	14.0	NA	NA	315
●★ Chocolate fudge bar, *Carnation Slender* (2 bars)	275	23.0	15.0	NA	NA	309
●★■ Chocolate mint bar, *Figurines* (2 bars)	275	21.0	16.0	NA	NA	175
●★ Chocolate peanut butter bar, *Carnation Slender* (2 bars)	275	24.0	15.0	NA	NA	294
★ Chocolate peanut butter granola bar, *Crunchola* (1 bar)	130	14.0	7.0	5.6	0	47
●★■ *Chocolate Susy Q's, Hostess* (1 cake)	240	36.0	9.0	NA	16	310
●★ Cinnamon bar, *Carnation Slender* (2 bars)	275	24.0	14.0	NA	NA	364
●★ Coconut macaroon bar, *Pepperidge Farm* (1 bar)	210	25.0	11.0	NA	NA	66
● Corn chips, *Planters* (1 oz.)	170	15.0	11.0	1.0	0	220
●★ Corn curls, *Flings Crispy* (1 oz.)	160	14.0	11.0	NA	NA	NA
●★ Crumb cake, *Hostess* (1 cake)	130	22.0	4.0	NA	10	95
●★■ Crunchy chocolate bar, *Figurines* (2 bars)	275	21.0	16.0	NA	NA	155
●★ Cupcake, chocolate, *Hostess* (1 cupcake)	160	30.0	5.0	NA	3	250
●★ Cupcake, orange, *Hostess* (1 cupcake)	150	27.0	4.0	NA	13	150

Alerts: ● Sodium ★ Sugar ■ Cholesterol

Food Description	Calories	Carbohydrates (grams)	Fat (grams)	Saturated Fat (grams)	Cholesterol (milligrams)	Sodium (milligrams)
●★ Date nut bar, *Pepperidge Farm* (1 bar)	160	29.0	5.0	NA	NA	52
●★ *Ding Dong, Hostess* (1 cake)	170	21.0	10.0	NA	6	95
●★ *Doo Dads* (1 oz.)	140	17.0	7.0	NA	NA	NA
●★■ Double chocolate bar, *Figurines* (2 bars)	275	21.0	16.0	NA	NA	130
●★ Food sticks, caramel, *Pillsbury* (4 sticks)	180	27.0	6.0	NA	NA	165
●★ Food sticks, chocolate mint, *Pillsbury* (4 sticks)	180	27.0	6.0	NA	NA	95
●★ Food sticks, chocolate, *Pillsbury* (4 sticks)	180	27.0	6.0	NA	NA	115
●★ Food sticks, orange, *Pillsbury* (4 sticks)	180	27.0	6.0	NA	NA	135
●★ Food sticks, peanut butter, *Pillsbury* (4 sticks)	180	27.0	6.0	NA	NA	160
●★ Granola bar, almond, *Nature Valley* (1 bar)	110	15.0	5.0	NA	0	80
●★ Granola bar, cinnamon, *Nature Valley* (1 bar)	110	16.0	4.0	NA	0	65
●★ Granola bar, coconut, *Nature Valley* (1 bar)	120	15.0	6.0	NA	0	60
●★ Granola bar, honey and oats, *Nature Valley* (1 bar)	110	16.0	4.0	NA	0	65
●★ Granola bar, peanut, *Nature Valley* (1 bar)	120	15.0	5.0	NA	0	80
●★ Granola clusters, almond, *Nature Valley* (1 roll)	140	27.0	3.0	NA	NA	140
●★ Granola clusters, caramel, *Nature Valley* (1 roll)	150	28.0	3.0	NA	NA	115
●★ Granola clusters, raisin, *Nature Valley* (1 roll)	140	28.0	2.0	NA	NA	120
●★ *Ho-Ho, Hostess* (1 cake)	120	17.0	6.0	NA	13	80
★■ Lemon yogurt bar, *Figurines* (2 bars)	275	21.0	16.0	NA	NA	45
● Nacho tortilla chips, *Planters* (1 oz.)	130	14.0	7.0	1.0	0	170
●★ Nut and snack mix, *Lipton Flavor Tree* (1 oz.)	160	10.0	12.0	NA	NA	NA
●★ Party mix, *Lipton Flavor Tree* (1 oz.)	160	10.0	11.0	NA	NA	NA
Popcorn						
Popped in oil, *TV Time* (1 cup)	70	7.0	4.0	NA	0	NA
Popped, large kernel (1 cup)	23	4.6	0.3	0	0	Tr.
● Popped, large kernel, with oil and salt (1 cup)	41	5.3	2.0	1.4	0	174

Alerts: ● Sodium ★ Sugar ■ Cholesterol

Food Description	Calories	Carbohydrates (grams)	Fat (grams)	Saturated Fat (grams)	Cholesterol (milligrams)	Sodium (milligrams)
★Popped, sugar coated (1 cup)	134	29.9	1.2	0.4	0	Tr.
Tender white, popped in oil, *3 Minute Super Pop* (1 quart)	220	20.0	15.0	NA	0	NA
Tender white, popped, *3 Minute Super Pop* (1 quart)	100	20.0	2.0	NA	0	10
Tender yellow, popped in oil, *3 Minute Super Pop* (1 quart)	220	20.0	15.0	NA	0	NA
Tender yellow, popped, *3 Minute Super Pop* (1 quart)	100	20.0	1.0	NA	0	10
Unpopped (1 cup)	742	147.8	9.6	1.0	0	6
Unsalted, popped, *Featherweight* (2¾ cups)	120	15.0	6.0	NA	0	7
●Potato chips (10 chips)	114	10.0	8.0	2.0	0	68
●Potato chips, *Planters* (1 oz.)	150	17.0	8.0	1.0	0	210
●Potato sticks (1 cup)	190	17.8	12.7	3.2	0	119
●Pretzels (1 Dutch type)	12	12.1	0.7	0.2	0	268
●Pretzels (10 3″ logs)	195	37.9	2.3	0.5	0	840
●Pretzels (10 rings)	78	15.2	0.9	0.2	0	336
●Pretzels (10 3″ sticks)	23	4.6	0.3	0.1	0	100
●Pretzels, Dutch, *Mister Salty* (1 oz.)	110	22.0	1.0	NA	0	NA
●Pretzels, little shapes, *Mister Salty* (1 oz.)	110	22.0	1.0	NA	0	NA
Pretzels, low sodium, *Featherweight* (3 pretzels)	20	4.0	0	0	0	5
●Pretzels, *Mister Salty* (0.9 oz.)	100	20.0	1.0	NA	0	NA
●Pretzels, sticks, *Mister Salty* (1 oz.)	110	22.0	1.0	NA	0	NA
●★Raisin spice bar, *Pepperidge Farm* (1 bar)	170	31.0	5.0	NA	NA	59
●★■Raspberry bar, *Figurines* (2 bars)	275	21.0	16.0	NA	NA	240
●★Sesame coconut crunch, *Lipton Flavor Tree* (1 oz.)	130	20.0	5.0	NA	NA	NA
●★Sesame honey crunch, *Lipton Flavor Tree* (1 oz.)	140	18.0	7.0	NA	NA	NA
●★*Sno Balls, Hostess* (1 cake)	140	25.0	4.0	NA	2	165
●★Sticks, cheddar, *Pepperidge Farm* (1 oz.)	120	19.0	5.0	NA	NA	370
●★Sticks, lightly salted, *Pepperidge Farm* (1 oz.)	120	18.0	4.0	NA	NA	300
●★Sticks, pumpernickel, *Pepperidge Farm* (1 oz.)	110	17.0	4.0	NA	NA	351
●★Sticks, sesame and bran, *Lipton Flavor Tree* (1 oz.)	160	11.0	11.0	NA	NA	NA

Alerts: ● Sodium ★ Sugar ■ Cholesterol

Food Description	Calories	Carbohydrates (grams)	Fat (grams)	Saturated Fat (grams)	Cholesterol (milligrams)	Sodium (milligrams)
●★Sticks, whole wheat, *Pepperidge Farm* (1 oz.)	110	17.0	4.0	NA	NA	366
★■Strawberry yogurt bar, *Figurines* (2 bars)	275	21.0	16.0	NA	NA	45
★Strawberry yogurt granola bar, *Crunchola* (1 bar)	120	15.0	6.0	4.5	0	32
●Taco tortilla chips, *Planters* (1 oz.)	130	14.0	7.0	1.0	0	170
●★■Tiger Tails, *Hostess* (2 cakes)	430	76.0	13.0	NA	51	480
●★■Twinkie, *Hostess* (1 cake)	140	26.0	4.0	NA	20	190
●★Vanilla bar, *Carnation Slender* (2 bars)	275	24.0	14.0	NA	NA	364
●★■Vanilla bar, *Figurines* (2 bars)	275	21.0	16.0	NA	NA	175

Soups and Broths

Food Description	Calories	Carbohydrates (grams)	Fat (grams)	Saturated Fat (grams)	Cholesterol (milligrams)	Sodium (milligrams)
●Bean with bacon, condensed, *Campbell's Manhandlers* (5½ oz.)	190	28.0	6.0	NA	NA	1020
●Bean with pork, condensed (11½ oz. can)	437	56.4	15.0	3.3	13	2627
●■Beef and country vegetables, *Campbell's Chunky* (10¾ oz.)	190	22.0	5.0	NA	NA	1035
■Beef and country vegetables, low sodium, ready to serve, *Campbell's Chunky* (7½ oz.)	170	16.0	6.0	NA	NA	70
●Beef and noodles, condensed, *Campbell's Broth Plus* (5 oz.)	80	10.0	3.0	NA	NA	910
●★Beef bouillon, *Maggi* (1 cube)	6	1.0	1.0	NA	NA	940
●Beef broth and barley, condensed, *Campbell's* (5½ oz.)	90	13.0	3.0	NA	NA	1100
●Beef broth and noodles, condensed, *Campbell's* (5 oz.)	80	10.0	3.0	NA	NA	910

Alerts: ● Sodium ★ Sugar ■ Cholesterol

Food Description	Calories	Carbohydrates (grams)	Fat (grams)	Saturated Fat (grams)	Cholesterol (milligrams)	Sodium (milligrams)
• Beef broth, condensed (10½ oz.)	77	6.6	0	0	57	1943
• Beef broth, condensed, *Campbell's* (5 oz.)	35	3.0	0	0	NA	1055
• Beef broth, condensed, *Campbell's Light Ones* (5 oz.)	30	2.0	0	0	NA	1055
• Beef, condensed, *Campbell's* (5½ oz.)	110	15.0	3.0	NA	NA	1120
• Beef consomme, condensed, *Campbell's* (5 oz.)	45	4.0	1.0	NA	NA	780
•★ Beef flavor bouillon, dry, *Herb-Ox* (1 cube)	6	1.0	1.0	NA	NA	NA
•★ Beef flavor bouillon, dry, *Wyler's* (1 cube)	1	1.0	1.0	NA	NA	NA
★ Beef flavor broth, dry, *Featherweight* (1 tsp.)	18	2.0	1.0	NA	NA	10
•★ Beef flavor noodle, prepared, *Cup-A-Soup* (6 oz.)	45	8.0	1.0	NA	NA	NA
•★ Beef flavor seasoned broth, *Herb-Ox* (1 packet)	8	1.0	0	0	NA	NA
• Beef mushroom, condensed, *Campbell's Light Ones* (5 oz.)	90	8.0	4.0	NA	NA	1220
•★ Beef mushroom, prepared, *Cup-A-Soup* (6 oz.)	40	7.0	1.0	NA	NA	NA
• Beef noodle, condensed (10½ oz.)	170	17.3	6.6	2.1	39	2276
• Beef noodle, condensed, *Campbell's Light Ones* (5 oz.)	90	9.0	3.0	NA	NA	1055
•★ Beef noodle, dehydrated (2 oz. package)	221	37.2	4.2	1.2	52	1350
•■ Beef noodle, stroganoff style, *Campbell's Chunky* (10¾ oz.)	280	24.0	14.0	NA	NA	1280
★ Beef soup base, *Featherweight* (1 tsp.)	20	3.0	1.0	NA	NA	7
• Beef vegetable with barley, condensed, *Campbell's Manhandlers* (5½ oz.)	110	15.0	3.0	NA	NA	NA
•★ Beefy onion, prepared, *Cup-A-Soup* (6 oz.)	30	4.0	1.0	NA	NA	NA
•★ Black bean, condensed, *Campbell's* (5½ oz.)	140	22.0	3.0	NA	NA	1410

Alerts: • Sodium ★ Sugar ■ Cholesterol

Food Description	Calories	Carbohydrates (grams)	Fat (grams)	Saturated Fat (grams)	Cholesterol (milligrams)	Sodium (milligrams)
•★ Black bean with sherry, canned, *Crosse & Blackwell* (6.5 oz.)	80	18.0	1.0	NA	NA	755
•★ Bouillon cube, instant (1 cube)	5	0.2	0.1	0	3	960
•★ Bouillon powder, instant (1 tsp.)	2	0.1	0.1	0	2	480
• Burly vegetable, semi-condensed, *Campbell's Soup for One* (7¾ oz.)	150	19.0	5.0	NA	NA	1445
•■ Cheddar cheese, condensed, *Campbell's* (5½ oz.)	180	14.0	11.0	NA	NA	1050
• Chicken alphabet, condensed, *Campbell's* (5 oz.)	110	14.0	3.0	NA	NA	1165
• Chicken and dumplings, condensed, *Campbell's* (5 oz.)	100	11.0	4.0	NA	NA	1075
• Chicken and rice, condensed, *Campbell's Broth Plus* (5 oz.)	60	8.0	3.0	NA	NA	1060
•★ Chicken and rice, prepared, *Cup-A-Soup* (6 oz.)	45	7.0	1.0	NA	NA	NA
• Chicken and stars, condensed, *Campbell's Light Ones* (5 oz.)	80	9.0	3.0	NA	NA	1150
• Chicken broth and noodles, condensed, *Campbell's* (5 oz.)	80	10.0	4.0	NA	NA	1140
• Chicken broth and vegetables, condensed, *Campbell's* (5 oz.)	30	4.0	1.0	NA	NA	1025
• Chicken broth, condensed, *Campbell's* (5 oz.)	50	3.0	2.0	NA	NA	980
• Chicken broth, condensed, *Campbell's Light Ones* (5 oz.)	50	4.0	3.0	NA	NA	980
• Chicken consomme, condensed (10½ oz.)	54	4.5	0.3	0	39	1794
•★ Chicken flavor bouillon, dry, *Herb-Ox* (1 cube)	6	1.0	1.0	NA	NA	NA
★ Chicken flavor broth, dry, *Featherweight* (1 tsp)	18	2.0	1.0	NA	NA	5
•★ Chicken flavor noodle, dry, prepared, *Mrs. Grass* (8 oz.)	73	11.0	1.0	NA	NA	NA
•★ Chicken flavor seasoned broth, *Herb-Ox* (1 packet)	12	2.0	0	0	NA	NA

Alerts: • Sodium ★ Sugar ■ Cholesterol

Food Description	Calories	Carbohydrates (grams)	Fat (grams)	Saturated Fat (grams)	Cholesterol (milligrams)	Sodium (milligrams)
●★ Chicken flavor seasoned broth, *Wyler's* (1 cube)	8	1.0	1.0	NA	NA	NA
●★ Chicken gumbo, condensed (10½ oz.)	137	18.2	3.9	0	36	2360
●★ Chicken gumbo, condensed, *Campbell's Light Ones* (5 oz.)	70	10.0	2.0	NA	NA	1090
●★ Chicken noodle and meat, prepared, *Cup-A-Soup* (6 oz.)	45	6.0	1.0	NA	NA	NA
★ Chicken noodle, canned, low sodium, *Campbell's* (7¼ oz.)	90	8.0	5.0	NA	NA	30
● Chicken noodle, condensed (10½ oz.)	158	19.7	4.8	0	39	2431
● Chicken noodle, condensed, *Campbell's* (5 oz.)	90	11.0	3.0	NA	7	1225
Chicken noodle, condensed, *Featherweight* (3¾ oz.)	60	8.0	2.0	NA	NA	50
● Chicken noodle, condensed, *Noodle-Os, Campbell's Light Ones* (5 oz.)	90	12.0	3.0	NA	NA	1105
●★ Chicken noodle, dehydrated (2 oz. package)	218	33.1	5.7	1.7	52	2438
●★ Chicken noodle with meat, prepared, *Cup-A-Soup* (6 oz.)	70	9.0	2.0	NA	NA	NA
● Chicken noodle with mushrooms, *Campbell's Chunky* (10¾ oz.)	230	22.0	8.0	NA	NA	1080
Chicken noodle with mushrooms, low sodium, ready to serve, *Campbell's Chunky* (7½ oz.)	160	14.0	6.0	NA	NA	80
●★ Chicken, prepared, *Cup-A-Broth* (6 oz.)	20	4.0	1.0	NA	NA	NA
●★ Chicken rice, prepared, *Cup-A-Soup* (6 oz.)	60	8.0	2.0	NA	NA	NA
● Chicken rice with country vegetables, *Campbell's Chunky* (9½ oz.)	150	15.0	4.0	NA	NA	1160
★ Chicken soup base, *Featherweight* (1 tsp.)	25	4.0	1.0	NA	NA	1
●★ Chicken Supreme, prepared, *Cup-A-Soup* (6 oz.)	90	11.0	3.0	NA	NA	NA

Aierts: ● Sodium ★ Sugar ■ Cholesterol

Food Description	Calories	Carbohydrates (grams)	Fat (grams)	Saturated Fat (grams)	Cholesterol (milligrams)	Sodium (milligrams)
• Chicken vegetable, *Campbell's Chunky* (9½ oz.)	190	21.0	5.0	NA	NA	1195
• Chicken vegetable, condensed (10½ oz.)	187	23.3	6.0	0	48	2551
• Chicken vegetable, condensed, *Campbell's Light Ones* (5 oz.)	90	10.0	4.0	NA	NA	1115
•★ Chicken vegetable, prepared, *Cup-A-Soup* (6 oz.)	40	7.0	1.0	NA	NA	NA
• Chicken vegetable, semi-condensed, *Campbell's Soup for One* (7¾ oz.)	130	14.0	6.0	NA	NA	1555
• Chicken with rice, condensed (10½ oz.)	116	14.0	3.0	0	36	2276
• Chicken with rice, condensed, *Campbell's Light Ones* (5 oz.)	80	9.0	3.0	NA	NA	990
•★ Chicken with rice, dehydrated (1½ oz. package)	152	27.0	2.9	0.8	45	1875
• Chili beef, condensed, *Campbell's Manhandlers* (5½ oz.)	180	23.0	6.0	NA	NA	1115
• Clam chowder, Manhattan style, *Campbell's Chunky* (9½ oz.)	160	23.0	4.0	NA	NA	1335
• Clam chowder, Manhattan style, canned, *Crosse & Blackwell* (6.5 oz.)	50	9.0	1.0	NA	NA	800
• Clam chowder, Manhattan style, condensed (10¾ oz.)	201	30.5	6.4	3.1	24	2336
• Clam chowder, Manhattan style, condensed, *Campbell's Light Ones* (5 oz.)	90	15.0	3.0	NA	NA	1030
• Clam chowder, New England, canned, *Crosse & Blackwell* (6.5 oz.)	90	14.0	3.0	NA	NA	635
• Clam chowder, New England, condensed, *Campbell's* (5 oz.)	100	13.0	3.0	NA	NA	1075
• Clam chowder, New England, semi-condensed, *Campbell's Soup for One* (7¾ oz.)	120	17.0	4.0	NA	NA	855

Alerts: • Sodium ★ Sugar ■ Cholesterol

Food Description	Calories	Carbohydrates (grams)	Fat (grams)	Saturated Fat (grams)	Cholesterol (milligrams)	Sodium (milligrams)
• Clear beef broth, *Swanson* (7¼ oz.)	20	1.0	1.0	NA	NA	765
• Clear chicken broth, *Swanson* (7¼ oz.)	35	1.0	2.0	NA	NA	780
• Consomme Madrilene, clear, canned, *Crosse & Blackwell* (6.5 oz.)	25	4.0	0	0	NA	1005
• Consomme Madrilene, red, canned, *Crosse & Blackwell* (6.5 oz.)	25	5.0	0	0	NA	1120
•★ Country vegetable, prepared, *Cup-A-Soup* (6 oz.)	80	14.0	1.0	NA	NA	NA
• Crab a la Maryland, canned, *Crosse & Blackwell* (6.5 oz.)	50	8.0	1.0	NA	NA	935
•★ Cream of asparagus, condensed (10½ oz.)	161	25.0	4.2	0	24	2443
•★ Cream of asparagus, condensed, *Campbell's* (5 oz.)	100	12.0	5.0	NA	NA	1160
• Cream of celery, condensed (10½ oz.)	215	22.1	12.5	2.2	18	2372
• Cream of celery, condensed, *Campbell's* (5 oz.)	120	10.0	9.0	NA	NA	1140
• Cream of chicken, condensed (10½ oz.)	235	20.0	14.3	2.3	24	2410
• Cream of chicken, condensed, *Campbell's* (5 oz.)	140	11.0	9.0	NA	NA	1225
•★ Cream of chicken, dry, prepared, *Mrs. Grass* (8 oz.)	69	10.0	0.9	NA	NA	NA
•★ Cream of chicken, instant, prepared, *Mrs. Grass* (6 oz.)	90	14.0	1.0	NA	NA	NA
•★ Cream of chicken, prepared, *Cup-A-Soup* (6 oz.)	80	10.0	3.0	NA	NA	NA
• Cream of mushroom bisque, canned, *Crosse & Blackwell* (6.5 oz.)	90	8.0	5.0	NA	NA	920
• Cream of mushroom, condensed (10½ oz. can)	331	25.0	23.8	3.3	24	2369
• Cream of mushroom, condensed, *Campbell's* (5 oz.)	120	11.0	8.0	NA	NA	990
★ Cream of mushroom, low sodium, condensed, *Featherweight* (4 oz.)	50	9.0	2.0	NA	NA	15

Alerts: • Sodium ★ Sugar ■ Cholesterol

Food Description	Calories	Carbohydrates (grams)	Fat (grams)	Saturated Fat (grams)	Cholesterol (milligrams)	Sodium (milligrams)
★ Cream of mushroom, low sodium, ready to serve, *Campbell's* (7¼ oz.)	140	10.0	10.0	NA	NA	35
●★ Cream of mushroom, prepared, *Cup-A-Soup* (6 oz.)	70	10.0	3.0	NA	NA	NA
● Cream of onion, condensed, *Campbell's* (5 oz.)	130	15.0	0.6	NA	NA	1065
● Cream of potato, condensed, *Campbell's* (5 oz.)	90	14.0	3.0	NA	NA	1115
●■ Cream of shrimp, canned, *Crosse & Blackwell* (6.5 oz.)	90	7.0	4.0	NA	NA	790
●■ Cream of shrimp, condensed, *Campbell's* (5 oz.)	110	10.0	8.0	NA	NA	1185
●★ Cream of vegetable, prepared, *Cup-A-Soup* (6 oz.)	80	12.0	3.0	NA	NA	NA
● Creamy chicken mushroom, condensed, *Campbell's* (5 oz.)	150	11.0	10.0	NA	NA	1340
● Curly noodle and chicken, condensed, *Campbell's* (5 oz.)	100	12.0	3.0	NA	NA	1135
●★ Gazpacho, canned, *Crosse & Blackwell* (6.5 oz.)	30	1.0	2.0	NA	NA	895
● Golden chicken noodle, semi-condensed, *Campbell's Chunky* (7¾ oz.)	130	14.0	5.0	NA	NA	1270
● Golden mushroom, condensed, *Campbell's* (5 oz.)	110	11.0	5.0	NA	NA	1135
● Green pea, condensed (11 oz.)	335	58.1	5.7	0	0	2319
● Green pea, condensed, *Campbell's* (5½ oz.)	210	34.0	4.0	NA	NA	990
●★ Green pea, dehydrated (4 oz. package)	409	69.6	4.6	1.7	0	2666
★ Green pea, low sodium, ready to serve, *Campbell's* (7½ oz.)	150	24.0	3.0	NA	NA	40
●★ Green pea, prepared, *Cup-A-Soup* (6 oz.)	100	19.0	1.0	NA	NA	NA
●★ Ham in butter bean, *Campbell's Chunky* (10¾ oz.)	290	31.0	12.0	NA	NA	1410
●★ Harvest vegetable, prepared, *Cup-A-Soup* (6 oz.)	100	20.0	1.0	Tr.	NA	NA

Alerts: ● Sodium ★ Sugar ■ Cholesterol

Food Description	Calories	Carbohydrates (grams)	Fat (grams)	Saturated Fat (grams)	Cholesterol (milligrams)	Sodium (milligrams)
•★Hearty chicken, prepared, *Cup-A-Soup* (6 oz.)	70	11.0	1.0	NA	NA	NA
• Mediterranean vegetable, canned, *Campbell's Chunky* (9½ oz.)	170	26.0	6.0	NA	NA	1520
• Minestrone, *Campbell's Chunky* (9½ oz.)	140	20.0	5.0	NA	NA	975
• Minestrone, canned, *Crosse & Blackwell* (6.5 oz.)	90	18.0	2.0	NA	NA	715
• Minestrone, condensed (10¾ oz.)	265	35.4	8.5	3.1	55	2479
• Minestrone, condensed, *Campbell's Manhandlers* (5 oz.)	90	13.0	3.0	NA	NA	1075
• Noodles and ground beef, condensed, *Campbell's Manhandlers* (5 oz.)	110	14.0	5.0	NA	NA	970
•★Noodles in chicken broth, instant, prepared, *Mrs. Grass* (6 oz.)	26	5.0	1.0	NA	NA	NA
•★Old fashioned bean and ham, *Campbell's Chunky* (11 oz.)	300	35.0	11.0	NA	NA	1148
•★Old-fashioned bean, semi-condensed, *Campbell's Soup for One* (7¾ oz.)	210	28.0	7.0	NA	NA	1110
•★Old fashioned tomato rice, condensed, *Campbell's* (5½ oz.)	150	29.0	3.0	NA	NA	835
• Old fashioned vegetable beef, *Campbell's Chunky* (9½ oz.)	160	19.0	5.0	NA	NA	852
• Old fashioned vegetable, condensed, *Campbell's Light Ones* (5 oz.)	90	13.0	3.0	NA	NA	1120
• Old world vegetable, semi-condensed, *Campbell's Soup for One* (7¾ oz.)	120	18.0	4.0	NA	NA	1205
• Onion, condensed (10½ oz.)	161	12.8	6.3	3.0	60	2607
• Onion, condensed, *Campbell's Light Ones* (5 oz.)	80	11.0	3.0	NA	NA	1245
•★Onion, dehydrated (1½ oz. package)	150	23.2	4.6	1.1	64	2870
•★Onion flavor seasoned broth, *Herb-Ox* (1 packet)	14	2.0	0	0	NA	NA

Alerts: • Sodium ★ Sugar ■ Cholesterol

Food Description	Calories	Carbohydrates (grams)	Fat (grams)	Saturated Fat (grams)	Cholesterol (milligrams)	Sodium (milligrams)
●★Onion mushroom, prepared, *Cup-A-Soup* (6 oz.)	40	6.0	1.0	NA	NA	NA
●★Onion, prepared, *Cup-A-Soup* (6 oz.)	20	3.0	1.0	NA	NA	NA
●★Oriental beef teriyaki, condensed, *Campbell's* (10 oz.)	90	11.0	2.0	NA	NA	1050
●★Oriental chicken, condensed, *Campbell's* (10 oz.)	70	6.0	4.0	NA	NA	1140
●Oriental won-ton, condensed, *Campbell's* (10 oz.)	50	6.0	2.0	NA	NA	1010
●■Oyster stew, condensed, *Campbell's* (5 oz.)	70	5.0	5.0	NA	NA	1000
●■Oyster stew, homemade, 1 part oysters, 2 parts milk (1 cup)	233	10.8	15.4	7.2	86	813
●Savory cream of mushroom, semi-condensed, *Campbell's Soup for One* (7½ oz.)	140	13.0	10.0	NA	NA	1285
●Scotch broth, condensed, *Campbell's Manhandlers* (5 oz.)	100	11.0	4.0	NA	NA	1050
●■Sirloin burger, *Campbell's Chunky* (10¾ oz.)	220	21.0	9.0	NA	NA	1140
●Spanish-style vegetable, condensed, *Campbell's* (10 oz.)	60	12.0	0	0	0	NA
●★Split pea, condensed (11¼ oz.)	376	54.2	8.3	2.7	13	2446
●★Split pea with ham and bacon, condensed, *Campbell's Manhandlers* (5½ oz.)	220	32.0	5.0	NA	NA	905
●★Split pea with ham, carrots, and potatoes, *Campbell's Chunky* (9½ oz.)	210	29.0	6.0	NA	NA	1200
●★Spring vegetable, prepared, *Cup-A-Soup* (6 oz.)	40	7.0	1.0	NA	NA	NA
●★Tomato bisque, condensed, *Campbell's* (5 oz.)	160	29.0	4.0	NA	NA	1150
●★Tomato, condensed (10¾ oz.)	220	38.7	6.4	1.1	0	2415
●★Tomato, condensed, *Campbell's* (5 oz.)	110	20.0	2.0	NA	4	1050
★Tomato, condensed, *Featherweight* (3¾ oz.)	60	13.0	0	0	0	26
●★Tomato garden, condensed, *Campbell's* (10 oz.)	100	23.0	0	0	0	NA

Alerts: ● Sodium ★ Sugar ■ Cholesterol

Food Description	Calories	Carbohydrates (grams)	Fat (grams)	Saturated Fat (grams)	Cholesterol (milligrams)	Sodium (milligrams)
★Tomato, low sodium, ready to serve, *Campbell's* (7¼ oz.)	140	23.0	4.0	NA	NA	40
●★Tomato, prepared, *Cup-A-Soup* (6 oz.)	80	17.0	1.0	NA	NA	NA
●★Tomato royale, semi-condensed, *Campbell's Soup for One* (7¾ oz.)	180	33.0	3.0	NA	NA	1130
●★Tomato vegetable with noodles, dehydrated (2½ oz. package)	247	44.5	5.7	1.5	0	4357
●Turkey and country vegetable, *Campbell's Chunky* (9¼ oz.)	140	15.0	5.0	NA	NA	1100
●Turkey noodle, condensed (10½ oz.)	194	20.9	7.2	2.1	57	2479
●Turkey noodle, condensed, *Campbell's Light Ones* (5 oz.)	80	10.0	3.0	NA	NA	1050
★Turkey noodle, low sodium, ready to serve, *Campbell's* (7¼ oz.)	60	7.0	3.0	NA	NA	55
●Turkey vegetable, condensed, *Campbell's Light Ones* (5 oz.)	90	10.0	4.0	NA	NA	980
●Vegetable and beef stockpot, condensed, *Campbell's* (5½ oz.)	120	20.0	2.0	NA	NA	1050
●Vegetable beef, condensed (10¾ oz.)	198	24.1	5.5	0	58	2604
●Vegetable beef, condensed, *Campbell's Light Ones* (5 oz.)	90	10.0	3.0	NA	NA	1135
●★Vegetable beef, dry, prepared, *Mrs. Grass* (8 oz.)	77	15.0	0.8	NA	NA	NA
Vegetable beef, low sodium, condensed, *Featherweight* (4 oz.)	80	12.0	3.0	NA	NA	15
Vegetable beef, low sodium, ready to serve, *Campbell's* (7¼ oz.)	90	8.0	3.0	NA	NA	60
●★Vegetable beef, prepared, *Cup-A-Soup* (6 oz.)	60	9.0	1.0	NA	NA	NA
●Vegetable, *Campbell's Chunky* (10¾ oz.)	140	24.0	4.0	NA	NA	1295
●Vegetable, condensed, *Campbell's* (5 oz.)	100	16.0	2.0	NA	NA	950

Alerts: ● Sodium ★ Sugar ■ Cholesterol

Food Description	Calories	Carbohydrates (grams)	Fat (grams)	Saturated Fat (grams)	Cholesterol (milligrams)	Sodium (milligrams)
★Vegetable, low sodium, ready to serve, *Campbell's* (7¼ oz.)	90	14.0	2.0	NA	NA	50
●Vegetables in beef broth, condensed (10¾ oz.)	195	33.6	4.3	0	27	2104
●Vegetarian vegetable, condensed (10¾ oz.)	195	32.3	5.2	0	0	2086
●Vegetarian vegetable, condensed, *Campbell's* (5 oz.)	90	16.0	2.0	NA	NA	820
●Vichyssoise, canned, *Crosse & Blackwell* (6.5 oz.)	70	5.0	4.0	NA	NA	700
●★Virginia pea, prepared, *Cup-A-Soup* (6 oz.)	140	18.0	5.0	NA	NA	NA

Sugars, Sweeteners, and Toppings

DESSERT TOPPINGS						
★Butterscotch flavor topping, *Smucker's* (2 Tbsp.)	140	33.0	0	0	0	NA
★Caramel flavor topping, *Smucker's* (2 Tbsp.)	140	33.0	0	0	0	NA
★Cherry topping, *Smucker's* (2 Tbsp.)	130	32.0	0	0	0	NA
★Chocolate flavor syrup, *Hershey* (2 Tbsp.)	80	17.0	1.0	NA	0	20
★Chocolate-flavored thin syrup or topping (1 oz.)	92	23.5	0.8	0.4	0	19
★Chocolate fudge syrup (1 oz.)	124	20.3	5.1	2.9	0	33
★Chocolate fudge topping, *Hershey* (2 Tbsp.)	100	14.0	4.0	NA	0	30
★Chocolate fudge topping, *Smucker's* (2 Tbsp.)	130	31.0	1.0	NA	0	NA
★Chocolate mint topping, *Smucker's* (2 Tbsp.)	140	31.0	1.0	NA	NA	NA
★Chocolate syrup, calorie reduced, *Featherweight* (1 Tbsp.)	30	7.0	0	0	0	NA

Alerts: ● Sodium ★ Sugar ■ Cholesterol

Food Description	Calories	Carbohydrates (grams)	Fat (grams)	Saturated Fat (grams)	Cholesterol (milligrams)	Sodium (milligrams)
★Peanut butter caramel topping, *Smucker's* (2 Tbsp.)	150	29.0	2.0	NA	0	NA
★Pecans-in-syrup topping, *Smucker's* (2 Tbsp.)	130	28.0	1.0	NA	0	NA
★Pineapple topping, *Smucker's* (2 Tbsp.)	130	32.0	0	0	0	NA
★Strawberry topping, *Smucker's* (2 Tbsp.)	120	30.0	0	0	0	NA
★Swiss milk chocolate fudge topping, *Smucker's* (2 Tbsp.)	140	31.0	NA	NA	0	NA
★Whipped topping, aerosol, *Lucky Whip* (2 Tbsp.)	25	1.0	2.3	1.5	NA	NA
★Whipped topping, *Featherweight* (2 Tbsp.)	1	1.0	0	0	0	NA
★Whipped topping, frozen, non-dairy, *Birds Eye Cool Whip* (1 Tbsp.)	14	1.0	1.0	NA	NA	1
Whipped topping mix, low calorie, *D-Zerta* (1 Tbsp.)	8	0	1.0	NA	NA	2
★Whipped topping mix, prepared, *Dream Whip* (1 Tbsp.)	8	1.0	0	0	NA	4
★Whipped topping mix, whipped, *Dieter's Gourmet* (1 Tbsp.)	8	1.0	1.0	NA	0	NA
SUGARS AND SWEETENERS						
Artificial sweetener, liquid, *Pillsbury Sweet 10* (⅛ tsp.)	0	0	0	0	0	1
Artificial sweetener, saccharin, *Featherweight* (¼ grain tablet)	0	0	0	0	0	2
Artificial sweetener, saccharin, *Featherweight* (½ grain tablet)	0	0	0	0	0	4
★Brown sugar, not packed (1 cup)	541	139.8	0	0	0	43
★Brown sugar, packed (1 cup)	821	212.1	0	0	0	66
Brown sugar substitute, *Sweet 'N Low* (¹⁄₁₀ tsp.)	2	0.5	0	0	0	NA
★Confectioner's sugar, sifted, *Domino* (¼ cup)	100	25.0	0	0	0	0
★Confectioner's sugar, unsifted, *Domino* (¼ cup)	120	30.0	0	0	0	0

Alerts: • Sodium ★ Sugar ■ Cholesterol

Food Description	Calories	Carbohydrates (grams)	Fat (grams)	Saturated Fat (grams)	Cholesterol (milligrams)	Sodium (milligrams)
★Fructose, granulated, *Estee* (1 tsp.)	15	4.0	0	0	0	0
★*Fructose Liquid Natural Sweetener, Sweet Lite* (½ tsp.)	10	3.0	0	0	0	0
★Fructose, *Sweet Lite Natural Sweetener* (1 packet)	11	3.0	0	0	0	Tr.
★Fructose, *Sweet Lite Natural Sweetener* (1 tsp.)	15	4.0	0	0	0	Tr.
★Granulated sugar (1 cup)	770	199.0	0	0	0	2
★Granulated sugar (1 tsp.)	15	4.0	0	0	0	0
★Granulated sugar (2 lumps)	19	5.0	0	0	0	Tr.
★Granulated sugar, *Domino* (1 level tsp.)	16	4.0	0	0	0	0
★Granulated sugar, *Domino Super Fine Bar Sugar* (1 level tsp.)	16	4.0	0	0	0	0
★Granulated sugar, with cinnamon, *Domino Sugar & Cinnamon* (1 gram)	6	1.0	0	0	0	0
★Honey (½ oz.)	43	11.5	0	0	0	Tr.
★Honey (1 cup)	1031	279.0	0	0	0	16
★Maple sugar (1 oz. piece)	99	25.5	0	0	0	4
★Molasses, blackstrap (1 cup)	699	180.4	0	0	0	314
★Molasses, *Grandma's Fancy* (1 Tbsp.)	57	NA	0	0	0	21
★Molasses, light (1 cup)	827	213.2	0	0	0	49
★Powdered sugar, sifted, spooned (1 cup)	385	99.5	0	0	0	1
★Powdered sugar, spooned (1 cup)	462	119.4	0	0	0	1
★Sugar cubes, *Domino Dots* (1 dot)	8	2.0	0	0	0	0
Sugar replacement, brown, *Sugar Twin* (1 tsp.)	2	0.4	0	0	0	2
Sugar replacement, granulated, *Sugar Twin* (1 tsp.)	2	0.4	0	0	0	2
Sugar replacement, granulated, *Sugar Twin* (1 packet)	3	0.8	0	0	0	2
Sugar substitute, granulated, *Sweet 'N Low* (1 packet)	4	1.0	0	0	0	4
Sugar substitute, granulated, *Sweet 'N Low* (1/10 tsp.)	2	0.5	0	0	0	NA

Alerts: ● Sodium ★ Sugar ■ Cholesterol

Food Description	Calories	Carbohydrates (grams)	Fat (grams)	Saturated Fat (grams)	Cholesterol (milligrams)	Sodium (milligrams)
Sugar substitute, liquid, concentrated, *Featherweight Sweetening* (3 drops)	0	0	0	0	0	1
Sugar substitute, *Pillsbury Sprinkle Sweet* (1 tsp.)	2	1.0	0	0	0	14
Sugar substitute, *Weight Watchers Sweet'ner* (1 packet)	4	1.0	0	0	0	NA
SYRUPS						
★Apricot syrup, *Smucker's* (2 Tbsp.)	100	26.0	0	0	0	NA
★Blackberry syrup, *Smucker's* (2 Tbsp.)	100	26.0	0	0	0	NA
★Blended syrup, cane and maple (1 cup)	794	204.8	0	0	0	6
★Blended syrup, cane and maple (1 Tbsp.)	50	12.8	0	0	0	Tr.
★Blended syrup, mainly corn (1 cup)	951	246.0	0	0	0	223
★Blended syrup, mainly corn (1 Tbsp.)	59	15.4	0	0	0	13
★Blueberry flavor glaze, bottled, *Solo* (2 oz.)	80	20.0	0.5	0	0	NA
●★Blueberry syrup, reduced calorie, *Featherweight* (1 Tbsp.)	14	3.0	0	0	0	NA
●★Corn syrup, dark, *Karo* (1 Tbsp.)	60	15.0	0	0	0	25
●★Corn syrup, light, *Karo* (1 Tbsp.)	60	15.0	0	0	0	25
★Grape syrup, *Smucker's* (2 Tbsp.)	100	26.0	0	0	0	NA
●★Imitation maple syrup, *Red Label* (1 tsp.)	4	1.0	0	0	0	NA
★Maple-honey flavor syrup, *Log Cabin* (1 Tbsp.)	50	15.0	0	0	0	3
★Maple syrup (1 cup)	794	204.8	0	0	0	31
★Maple syrup (1 Tbsp.)	50	12.8	0	0	0	2
●★Maple syrup, buttered, *Log Cabin* (1 Tbsp.)	60	14.0	0	0	1	30
★Maple syrup, *Log Cabin* (1 Tbsp.)	50	13.0	0	0	0	5
★Maple syrup, *Log Cabin Country Kitchen Maple* (1 Tbsp.)	50	13.0	0	0	0	5

Alerts: ● Sodium ★ Sugar ■ Cholesterol

Food Description	Calories	Carbohydrates (grams)	Fat (grams)	Saturated Fat (grams)	Cholesterol (milligrams)	Sodium (milligrams)
●★Maple syrup, *Mrs. Butterworth's* (3 Tbsp.)	160	39.0	0.9	0.4	5	NA
★Pancake and waffle syrup, imitation maple, *Karo* (1 Tbsp.)	60	15.0	0	0	0	20
★Pancake and waffle syrup, maple, *Golden Griddle* (1 Tbsp.)	50	13.5	0	0	NA	15
★Pancake and waffle syrup, maple, *Karo* (1 Tbsp.)	60	15.0	0	0	0	20
●★Pancake syrup, reduced calorie, *Featherweight* (1 Tbsp.)	12	3.0	0	0	0	NA
★Peach flavor glaze, bottled, *Solo* (2 oz.)	80	20.0	0.5	0	0	NA
★Strawberry flavor glaze, bottled, *Solo* (2 oz.)	80	20.0	0.5	0	0	NA
★Strawberry syrup, *Smucker's* (2 Tbsp.)	100	26.0	0	0	0	NA
●★Syrup product, *Aunt Jemima Lite* (1 oz.)	60	15.0	0	0	0	NA
★Sorghum syrup (1 cup)	848	224.4	0	0	0	33
★Sorghum syrup (1 Tbsp.)	53	14.0	0	0	0	2

Vegetables

Food Description	Calories	Carbohydrates (grams)	Fat (grams)	Saturated Fat (grams)	Cholesterol (milligrams)	Sodium (milligrams)
Acorn squash, baked, without salt (½ squash)	86	21.8	0.2	0	0	2
Acorn squash, baked, without salt, mashed (1 cup)	113	28.7	0.2	0	0	2
Acorn squash, boiled, without salt, mashed (1 cup)	83	20.6	0.2	0	0	2
Artichoke, globe or French, boiled, without salt, drained (1 medium bud)	45	11.9	0.2	0	0	36
Artichoke hearts, frozen, *Birds Eye* (3 oz.)	20	5.0	0	0	0	40
Asparagus						
Boiled, without salt, drained (4 medium spears)	12	2.2	0.1	0	0	Tr.

Alerts: ● Sodium ★ Sugar ■ Cholesterol

Food Description	Calories	Carbohydrates (grams)	Fat (grams)	Saturated Fat (grams)	Cholesterol (milligrams)	Sodium (milligrams)
Canned, *Larsen* (1 cup)	50	7.0	0	0	0	10
Canned, low sodium, *Featherweight* (½ cup)	20	3.0	0	0	0	10
Canned, low sodium, *Nutradiet* (½ cup)	17	3.0	0	0	0	10
● Cut, canned, *Stokely-Van Camp* (1 cup)	40	6.0	1.0	NA	0	690
Cut, frozen, *Birds Eye* (3.3 oz.)	25	3.0	0	0	0	3
● Green spears and tips, canned, *Del Monte* (1 cup)	35	6.0	1.0	NA	0	855
Pieces, boiled, without salt, drained (1 cup)	29	5.2	0.3	0	0	1
● Spears, canned, *Green Giant* (3½ oz.)	15	1.7	0.1	0	0	362
Spears, frozen, *Birds Eye* (3.3 oz.)	25	3.0	0	0	0	2
Spears, frozen, *Stokely-Van Camp* (2.6 oz.)	20	3.0	0	0	0	15
Spears, frozen, *Winter Garden* (2⅔ oz.)	18	3.0	0	0	0	5
Bamboo shoots, pieces, raw (8 oz.)	61	11.8	0.7	0	0	11
● Bean sprouts, canned, drained, *La Choy* (3½ oz.)	10	1.0	0.1	Tr.	0.1	71
Beets						
Boiled, without salt, drained, diced or sliced (1 cup)	54	12.2	0.2	0	0	73
●★ Canned, *Larsen* (1 cup)	100	20.0	0	0	NA	120
●★ Diced, canned, *Stokely-Van Camp* (1 cup)	70	15.0	0	0	0	525
●★ Pickled, crinkle cut, canned, *Del Monte* (1 cup)	150	36.0	0	0	0	665
●★ Pickled, sliced, canned, *Aunt Nellie's* (1 cup)	230	51.0	1	NA	NA	NA
●★ Pickled, sliced, canned, *Stokely-Van Camp* (1 cup)	180	45.0	0	0	0	565
●★ Sliced, canned, *Del Monte* (1 cup)	70	15.0	0	0	0	585
★ Sliced, canned, *Featherweight* (½ cup)	45	10.0	0	0	0	55
●★ Sliced, canned, *Libby* (1 cup)	70	16.0	0	0	0	NA
★ Sliced, canned, low sodium, *Nutradiet* (½ cup)	35	9.0	0	0	0	40
●★ Tiny whole, canned, *Aunt Nellie's* (1 cup)	80	18.0	0	0	0	NA

Alerts: ● Sodium ★ Sugar ■ Cholesterol

Food Description	Calories	Carbohydrates (grams)	Fat (grams)	Saturated Fat (grams)	Cholesterol (milligrams)	Sodium (milligrams)
●★ Whole, canned, *Del Monte* (1 cup)	70	15.0	0	0	0	585
●★ Whole, canned, *Stokely-Van Camp* (1 cup)	90	20.0	0	0	0	495
● Beet greens, boiled, without salt, drained (1 cup)	26	4.8	0.3	0	0	110
●★ Black-eye peas, frozen, *Green Giant Southern Recipe* (3½ oz.)	112	13.5	4.2	NA	NA	610
★ Black-eye peas, frozen, *Winter Garden* (3.3 oz.)	130	23.0	1.0	NA	NA	6
Black-eye peas, immature seeds, boiled, without salt, drained (1 cup)	178	29.9	1.3	0	0	2
● Black-eye peas, immature seeds, canned, with liquid (1 cup)	179	31.6	0.8	0	0	601
Broccoli						
Baby spears, frozen, *Birds Eye* (3.3 oz.)	25	4.0	0	0	0	15
Chopped, frozen, *Birds Eye* (3.3 oz.)	25	4.0	0	0	0	15
Chopped, frozen, *Stokely-Van Camp* (3.3 oz.)	25	4.0	0	0	0	20
Florets, frozen, *Winter Garden* (3.3 oz.)	25	5.0	0	0	0	NA
Pieces, boiled, without salt, drained (1 cup)	40	7.0	0.5	0	0	15
Spears, frozen, *Stokely-Van Camp* (3.3 oz.)	30	5.0	0	0	0	15
Spears, frozen, *Winter Garden* (3.3 oz.)	25	5.0	0	0	0	16
Brussels Sprouts						
Baby, frozen, *Birds Eye* (3.3 oz.)	35	6.0	0	0	0	5
Boiled, without salt, drained (1 cup)	56	9.9	0.6	0	0	15
Frozen, *Birds Eye* (3.3 oz.)	30	5.0	0	0	0	4
Frozen, *Stokely-Van Camp* (3.3 oz.)	35	7.0	0	0	0	10
Frozen, *Winter Garden* (3.3 oz.)	35	7.0	0	0	0	13
●★ With butter sauce, frozen, *Green Giant* (3½ oz.)	56	5.3	2.5	NA	NA	458

Alerts: ● Sodium ★ Sugar ■ Cholesterol

Food Description	Calories	Carbohydrates (grams)	Fat (grams)	Saturated Fat (grams)	Cholesterol (milligrams)	Sodium (milligrams)
Butternut squash, baked, without salt, mashed (1 cup)	139	35.9	0.2	0	0	2
Butternut squash, boiled, without salt, mashed (1 cup)	100	25.5	0.2	0	0	3
Cabbage, Chinese (pe-tsai), pieces (1 cup)	10	2.3	0.1	0	0	17
Cabbage, green, wedges, boiled, no salt, drained (1 cup)	31	6.8	0.3	0	0	22
Cabbage, green, sliced or coarsely shredded (1 cup)	17	3.8	0.1	0	0	14
Cabbage, red, sliced or coarsely shredded (1 cup)	22	4.8	0.1	0	0	18
Cabbage, savoy, sliced or coarsely shredded (1 cup)	17	3.2	0.1	0	0	15
Carrots						
Carrot (1 large)	30	7.0	0.1	0	0	33
★Canned, *Larsen* (1 cup)	70	15.0	0	0	0	60
★Crinkle sliced, frozen, *Winter Garden* (3.2 oz.)	40	9.0	0	0	0	42
★Cut frozen, *Stokely-Van Camp* (3 oz.)	30	7.0	0	0	0	30
●★Diced, canned, *Stokely-Van Camp* (1 cup)	50	12.0	0	0	0	620
Grated or shredded (1 cup)	46	10.7	0.2	0	0	51
Sliced, boiled, without salt, drained (1 cup)	48	11.0	0.3	0	0	51
●★Sliced, canned, *Del Monte* (1 cup)	60	14.0	0	0	0	565
★Sliced, canned, low sodium, *Featherweight* (½ cup)	30	6.0	0	0	0	30
★Sliced, canned, low sodium, *Nutradiet* (½ cup)	30	7.0	0	0	0	50
●★Sliced, canned, *Stokely-Van Camp* (1 cup)	45	10.0	0	0	0	520
Cauliflower, boiled, without salt, drained (1 cup)	28	5.1	0.3	0	0	11
Cauliflower, florets, frozen, *Winter Garden* (3.2 oz.)	25	4.0	0	0	0	18
Cauliflower, frozen, *Birds Eye* (3.3 oz.)	25	4.0	0	0	0	10
Cauliflower, frozen, *Stokely-Van Camp* (3.3 oz.)	25	5.0	0	0	0	15
●Celery (1 lb.)	68	15.3	0.4	0	0	509
●Celery (3 small inner stalks)	9	1.9	0.1	0	0	63

Alerts: ● Sodium ★ Sugar ■ Cholesterol

Food Description	Calories	Carbohydrates (grams)	Fat (grams)	Saturated Fat (grams)	Cholesterol (milligrams)	Sodium (milligrams)
• Celery, chopped or diced (1 cup)	20	4.7	0.1	0	0	151
Chicory, chopped (1 cup)	13	2.9	0.1	0	0	6
Collard greens (1 lb.)	204	34.0	3.6	0	0	195
Collard greens, boiled, without salt, drained (1 cup)	63	9.7	1.3	0	0	47
Collard greens, chopped, frozen, *Birds Eye* (3.3 oz.)	25	4.0	0	0	0	45
Collards, chopped, frozen, *Winter Garden* (3.3 oz.)	25	5.0	0	0	0	14
Corn						
★ Canned, *Larsen* (1 cup)	210	45.0	1.0	NA	NA	15
•★ Canned, *Libby* (1 cup)	160	37.0	2.0	NA	0	600
•★ Cream style, canned, *Green Giant* (3½ oz.)	85	18.5	0.5	NA	NA	287
•★ Cream style, canned, *Libby* (1 cup)	170	42.0	2.0	NA	0	530
★ Cream style, canned, low sodium, *Nutradiet* (½ cup)	80	15.0	1.0	NA	0	10
★ Cut, frozen, *Winter Garden* (3.3 oz.)	80	20.0	1.0	NA	0	4
•★ Golden, cream style, canned, *Stokely-Van Camp* (1 cup)	210	47.0	1.0	NA	0	765
•★ Golden, liquid pack, canned, *Stokely-Van Camp* (1 cup)	180	39.0	1.0	NA	0	620
On the cob, boiled, without salt (1 ear)	70	16.2	0.8	0	0	0
★ On the cob, frozen, *Birds Eye* (1 ear)	130	28.0	1.0	NA	0	3
★ On the cob, frozen, *Green Giant Niblets Ears* (1 ear)	160	33.0	1.0	NA	0	14
★ On the cob, frozen, *Ore-Ida* (4.5 oz.)	140	27.0	1.0	0	0	10
•★ White, canned, *Green Giant* (3½ oz.)	85	17.5	0.5	0	0	230
•★ White, cream style, canned, *Stokely-Van Camp* (1 cup)	200	47.0	1.0	NA	NA	730
★ Whole kernel, canned, low sodium, *Featherweight* (½ cup)	80	16.0	1.0	0	0	10
•★ Whole kernel, canned, *Del Monte* (1 cup)	150	36.0	1.0	NA	0	635
•★ Whole kernel, canned, *Green Giant Niblets* (3½ oz.)	83	17.2	0.5	0	0	281
★ Whole kernel, frozen, *Birds Eye 5 Minute* (3.3 oz.)	70	18.0	0	0	0	2

Alerts: • Sodium ★ Sugar ■ Cholesterol

Food Description	Calories	Carbohydrates (grams)	Fat (grams)	Saturated Fat (grams)	Cholesterol (milligrams)	Sodium (milligrams)
●★With butter sauce, frozen, *Green Giant Niblets* (3½ oz.)	93	15.1	2.6	NA	NA	331
Cress, garden (1 lb.)	145	24.9	3.2	0	0	63
Cress, garden, boiled briefly, without salt, drained (1 cup)	31	5.1	0.8	0	0	10
Crookneck or straightneck squash, cubed, boiled, without salt, drained (1 cup)	31	6.5	0.4	0	0	2
Crookneck squash, sliced, frozen, *Winter Garden* (3.3 oz.)	18	4.0	0	0	0	2
Cucumbers, pared, sliced (1 cup)	20	4.5	0	0	0	8
Dandelion greens (1 lb.)	204	41.7	3.2	0	0	344
Eggplant, boiled, no salt, drained (1 lb.)	86	18.6	0.9	0	0	5
Eggplant, diced, boiled, without salt, drained (1 cup)	38	8.2	0.4	0	0	2
Endive and escarole (1 lb.)	91	18.6	0.5	0	0	63
Green Beans						
Canned, low sodium, *Nutradiet* (½ cup)	20	4.0	0	0	0	10
French style, canned, *Featherweight* (½ cup)	25	5.0	0	0	0	10
●French style, canned, *Green Giant* (3½ oz.)	30	6.0	0.1	0	0	359
●French style, canned, *Libby* (1 cup)	35	8.0	0	0	0	685
French style, frozen, *Winter Garden* (3.2 oz.)	25	6.0	0	0	0	3
Pieces, boiled, without salt (1 cup)	31	6.8	0.3	0	0	5
●Pieces, boiled, with salt (1 cup)	31	6.8	0.3	0	0	300
●Pieces, canned, *Del Monte* (1 cup)	40	8.0	0	0	0	895
●Pieces, canned, *Libby* (1 cup)	40	8.0	0	0	0	685
Pieces, canned, low sodium, *Featherweight* (½ cup)	25	5.0	0	0	0	10
Pieces, frozen, *Birds Eye* (3 oz.)	25	5.0	0	0	0	2
●Pieces, with butter sauce, frozen, *Green Giant* (3½ oz.)	38	3.5	2.1	NA	NA	420
●Sliced, canned, *Stokely-Van Camp* (1 cup)	35	8.0	0	0	0	910

Alerts: ● Sodium ★ Sugar ■ Cholesterol

Food Description	Calories	Carbohydrates (grams)	Fat (grams)	Saturated Fat (grams)	Cholesterol (milligrams)	Sodium (milligrams)
• Whole, canned, *Del Monte* (1 cup)	35	6.0	0	0	0	925
• Whole, canned, *Stokely-Van Camp* (1 cup)	30	7.0	0	0	0	910
Green onions, whole (1 lb.)	163	37.2	0.9	0	0	22
Hubbard squash, baked, without salt (1 lb.)	227	53.1	1.8	0	0	5
Hubbard squash, baked, without salt, mashed (1 cup)	103	24.0	0.8	0	0	2
Hubbard squash, cubed, boiled, without salt (1 cup)	71	16.2	0.7	0	0	2
•★ Italian beans, canned, *Del Monte* (1 cup)	60	11.0	0	0	0	965
Kale, chopped, frozen, *Birds Eye* (3.3 oz.)	25	5.0	0	0	0	15
Kale, leaf, cut, frozen, *Winter Garden* (3.3 oz.)	25	5.0	0	0	0	14
Kale, leaves (1 lb.)	240	40.8	3.6	0	0	340
Kale, leaves, boiled, without salt, drained (1 cup)	43	6.7	0.8	0	0	47
Kohlrabi, diced, boiled, without salt, drained (1 cup)	40	8.7	0.2	0	0	10
Lettuce, Boston or Bibb, pieces (1 cup)	8	1.4	0.1	0	0	5
Lettuce, Iceberg (6″ head)	70	15.6	0.5	0	0	48
Lettuce, Iceberg, chunks (1 cup)	10	2.2	0.1	0	0	7
Lettuce, Romaine or Cos (1 lb.)	82	15.9	1.4	0	0	40
Lima Beans						
• Baby, frozen, *Winter Garden* (3.3 oz.)	130	24.0	0	0	0	165
• Canned, *Del Monte* (1 cup)	150	29.0	1.0	NA	0	685
Canned, *Featherweight* (½ cup)	80	16.0	0	0	0	25
• Fordhook, frozen, *Winter Garden* (3.3 oz.)	100	18.0	0	0	0	NA
• Immature, baby, frozen (10 oz. package)	346	65.3	0.6	0	0	417
Immature, boiled, without salt, drained (1 cup)	189	33.7	0.8	0	0	2
Immature, canned, low sodium, drained (1 cup)	162	30.1.	0.5	0	0	7
• Seasoned, canned, *Del Monte* (1 cup)	160	29.0	1.0	NA	0	685

Alerts: • Sodium ★ Sugar ■ Cholesterol

Food Description	Calories	Carbohydrates (grams)	Fat (grams)	Saturated Fat (grams)	Cholesterol (milligrams)	Sodium (milligrams)
Mung beans, seeds (1 cup)	714	126.6	2.7	0	0	12
Mung beans, sprouts, boiled, without salt, drained (1 cup)	35	6.5	0.3	0	0	5
Mushrooms (1 lb.)	127	20.0	1.4	0	0	68
Mushrooms, pieces (1 cup)	20	3.1	0.2	0	0	11
• Mushrooms, sliced, canned, *Green Giant* (3½ oz.)	23	3.0	0.2	0	0	467
• Mushrooms, with butter sauce, frozen, *Green Giant* (3½ oz.)	52	3.0	3.5	NA	NA	210
Mustard greens (1 lb.)	141	25.4	2.3	0	0	145
Mustard greens, boiled, without salt, drained (1 cup)	32	5.6	0.6	0	0	25
Mustard greens, chopped, frozen, *Birds Eye* (3.3 oz.)	20	3.0	0	0	0	25
Mustard greens, chopped, frozen, *Winter Garden* (3.3 oz.)	20	3.0	0	0	0	27
• New Zealand spinach (1 lb.)	86	14.1	1.4	0	0	721
• New Zealand spinach, boiled, without salt, drained (1 cup)	23	3.8	0.4	0	0	165
Okra, cut, frozen, *Birds Eye* (3.3 oz.)	25	6.0	0	0	0	3
Okra, sliced, boiled, without salt, drained (1 cup)	46	9.6	0.5	0	0	3
Okra, sliced, frozen (10 oz. package)	111	25.6	0.3	0	0	6
Okra, whole, frozen, *Winter Garden* (3.3 oz.)	30	7.0	0	0	0	3
Onions, boiled, without salt, drained (1 cup)	61	13.6	0.2	0	0	14
Onions, chopped, frozen, *Birds Eye* (1 oz.)	8	2.0	0	0	0	2
Onions, chopped, frozen, *Ore-Ida* (2 oz.)	20	4.0	0	0	0	10
Onions, sliced (1 cup)	44	10.0	0.1	0	0	11
Onions, small whole, frozen, *Birds Eye* (4 oz.)	40	10.0	0	0	NA	10
Parsnips, diced, boiled, without salt, drained (1 cup)	102	23.1	0.8	0	0	12
Peas						
★ Canned, *Larsen* (1 cup)	90	20.0	0	0	0	10
★ Crowder, frozen, *Winter Garden* (3.2 oz.)	130	23.0	1.0	NA	NA	5
• ★ Early, canned, *Stokely-Van Camp* (1 cup)	120	25.0	1.0	NA	0	740

Alerts: • Sodium ★ Sugar ■ Cholesterol

Food Description	Calories	Carbohydrates (grams)	Fat (grams)	Saturated Fat (grams)	Cholesterol (milligrams)	Sodium (milligrams)
Green, boiled, without salt, drained (1 cup)	114	19.4	0.6	0	0	2
•★Green, canned, *LeSueur* (1 cup)	110	19.0	1.0	NA	0	310
★Green, canned, low sodium, *Featherweight* (½ cup)	70	12.0	0	0	0	10
•★Green, early, canned, *Del Monte* (1 cup)	120	22.0	1.0	NA	0	670
•★Green, frozen, *Birds Eye 5 Minute* (3.3 oz.)	70	12.0	0	0	0	110
•★Green, frozen, *Winter Garden* (3.3 oz.)	80	13.0	1.0	NA	NA	93
•★Seasoned, canned, *Del Monte* (1 cup)	120	25.0	1.0	NA	0	605
•★Sweet, canned, *Green Giant Small Sweetlets* (3½ oz.)	40	6.8	0.3	0	0	280
•★Sweet, canned, *Libby* (1 cup)	120	23.0	1.0	NA	0	645
★Sweet, canned, low sodium, *Nutradiet* (½ cup)	40	8.0	0	0	0	10
•★Sweet, canned, *Stokely-Van Camp* (1 cup)	120	24.0	1.0	NA	0	600
•★Sweet, small, canned, *Freshlike* (1 cup)	120	20.0	1.0	NA	0	NA
•★Sweet, with butter sauce, frozen, *Green Giant* (3½ oz.)	79	9.2	2.9	NA	NA	425
Peppers, sweet, green (1 lb.)	100	21.8	0.9	0	0	59
Peppers, sweet, green, diced (1 cup)	33	7.2	0.3	0	0	19
Peppers, sweet, red (1 lb.)	141	32.2	1.4	0	0	59
Pimientos, canned, with liquid (2 oz.)	15	3.3	0.3	0	0	14
Potatoes						
Baked, without salt (7 oz.)	145	32.8	0.2	0	0	6
Boiled in skin, without salt (5 oz.)	104	23.3	0.1	0	0	4
★Cottage fries, frozen, *Birds Eye* (2.8 oz.)	120	17.0	5.0	NA	0	15
★Cottage fries, frozen, *Ore-Ida* (3 oz.)	140	22.0	5.0	3.0	0	30
•★Crinkle fries, frozen, *Carnation* (3½ oz.)	150	23.0	5.0	NA	0	58
★Crinkles, frozen, *Ore-Ida* (3 oz.)	130	21.0	5.0	3.0	0	25
★Dinner fries, frozen, *Ore-Ida* (3 oz.)	120	18.0	5.0	2.0	0	30

Alerts: • Sodium ★ Sugar ■ Cholesterol

Food Description	Calories	Carbohydrates (grams)	Fat (grams)	Saturated Fat (grams)	Cholesterol (milligrams)	Sodium (milligrams)
French fried, without salt (10 medium fries)	137	18.0	6.6	1.7	0	3
★French fries, frozen, *Birds Eye* (3 oz.)	110	17.0	4.0	NA	0	25
●Fried, with salt (1 cup)	456	55.4	24.1	6.0	0	379
★Hash browns, frozen, *Ore-Ida* (6 oz.)	120	24.0	0	0	0	35
★Hash browns, shredded, frozen, *Birds Eye* (3 oz.)	60	13.0	0	0	0	40
●★Hash browns, Southern style, frozen, *Carnation* (3½ oz.)	180	24.0	6.0	NA	NA	71
●★Hash browns, Southern style, with butter sauce, *Ore-Ida* (3 oz.)	120	15.0	6.0	5.0	5	60
●Hash browns, with salt (1 cup)	355	45.1	18.1	4.5	0	446
Mashed, flakes, dry (1 cup)	164	37.8	0.3	0	0	40
●Mashed, with milk and salt added (1 cup)	137	27.3	1.5	0	4	632
●New, canned, *Del Monte* (1 cup)	90	19.0	0	0	0	850
New, whole, frozen, *Winter Garden* (3.2 oz.)	60	13.0	0	0	0	6
Pared, boiled, without salt (5 oz.)	88	19.6	0.1	0	0	3
★Self-sizzling fries, frozen, *Heinz* (3 oz.)	160	24.0	9.0	4.0	0	30
★Shoestrings, frozen, *Ore-Ida* (3 oz.)	170	22.0	7.0	4.0	0	40
●Slices, with butter sauce, frozen, *Green Giant* (3½ oz.)	80	11.6	3.3	NA	NA	395
★Steak fries, frozen, *Birds Eye* (3 oz.)	110	18.0	3.0	NA	0	25
●★*Tasti Puffs,* frozen, *Birds Eye* (2.5 oz.)	190	19.0	12.0	NA	NA	400
●★*Taters,* frozen, *Carnation* (3½ oz.)	190	29.0	7.0	NA	0	70
●★*Tater Tots,* plain, frozen, *Ore-Ida* (3 oz.)	160	20.0	7.0	4.0	0	600
●Whole, canned, *Stokely-Van Camp* (1 cup)	100	21.0	1.0	NA	0	590
Whole, peeled, frozen, *Birds Eye* (3.2 oz.)	60	13.0	0	0	0	5
Pumpkin, canned, *Del Monte* (1 cup)	80	18.0	1.0	NA	0	15
Pumpkin, canned, *Libby* (1 cup)	80	20.0	1.0	NA	0	10

Alerts: ● Sodium ★ Sugar ■ Cholesterol

Food Description	Calories	Carbohydrates (grams)	Fat (grams)	Saturated Fat (grams)	Cholesterol (milligrams)	Sodium (milligrams)
●★Pumpkin, pie filling, canned, *Libby* (1 cup)	210	56.0	0	0	0	420
●★Pumpkin, pie filling, *Stokely-Van Camp* (1 cup)	350	87.0	0	0	0	840
Radishes, without tops (6 oz.)	26	5.5	0.2	0	0	27
Rutabagas, cubed, boiled, without salt, drained (1 cup)	60	13.9	0.2	0	0	7
Salsify, cubed, boiled, without salt, drained (1 cup)	94	20.4	0.8	0	0	12
●Sauerkraut, canned, *Del Monte* (1 cup)	50	11.0	0	0	0	1470
●Sauerkraut, chopped, canned, *Stokely-Van Camp* (1 cup)	40	9.0	0	0	0	1820
●Sauerkraut, drained, bottled, *Oscar Mayer* (½ cup)	15	2.8	0.2	0	0	505
Scallop squash, cubed, boiled, without salt, drained (1 cup)	34	8.0	0.2	0	0	2
Shallot bulb, chopped (1 Tbsp.)	7	1.7	0	0	0	2
Soybean sprouts (1 cup)	48	5.6	1.5	0	0	5
Soybean sprouts, boiled, without salt, drained (1 cup)	48	4.6	1.7	0	0	5
Spinach						
Boiled, without salt, drained (1 cup)	41	6.5	0.5	0	0	90
●Canned, *Del Monte* (1 cup)	45	8.0	1.0	NA	0	745
Canned, *Featherweight* (½ cup)	35	4.0	1.0	NA	0	35
Canned, *Larsen* (1 cup)	45	7.0	0	0	0	25
Chopped (1 cup)	14	2.4	0.2	0	0	39
Chopped, frozen, *Birds Eye* (3.3 oz.)	20	3.0	0	0	0	45
●Chopped, frozen, *Stokely-Van Camp* (3.3 oz.)	25	4.0	0	0	0	70
●Leaf, cut, frozen, *Winter Garden* (3.2 oz.)	25	4.0	0	0	0	74
●Leaf, frozen, *Stokely-Van Camp* (3.3 oz.)	25	4.0	0	0	0	70
●Leaves, cut, with butter sauce, frozen, *Green Giant* (3½ oz.)	44	2.5	2.7	NA	NA	360
★Squash, cooked, frozen, *Winter Garden* (3 oz.)	45	11.0	0	0	0	3
★Squash, frozen, *Stokely-Van Camp* (4 oz.)	45	10.0	0	0	0	10

Alerts: ● Sodium ★ Sugar ■ Cholesterol

Food Description	Calories	Carbohydrates (grams)	Fat (grams)	Saturated Fat (grams)	Cholesterol (milligrams)	Sodium (milligrams)
Summer squash, cubed, boiled, without salt, drained (1 cup)	29	6.5	0.2	0	0	2
★Summer squash, sliced, frozen, *Birds Eye* (3.3 oz.)	18	4.0	0	0	0	1
Sweet potato, baked, without salt (5″ potato)	162	37.0	0.6	0	0	14
Sweet potatoes, boiled, without salt, mashed (1 cup)	291	67.1	1.0	0	0	26
★Sweet potato, candied, homemade (½ medium)	176	35.9	3.5	1.7	9	44
●★Sweet potatoes, candied, orange, frozen, *Mrs. Paul's* (4 oz.)	180	44.0	0	0	0	240
●★Sweet potatoes, pieces, canned, with liquid (1 cup)	216	49.8	0.4	0	0	96
● Swiss chard, boiled, without salt, drained (1 cup)	26	4.8	0.3	0	0	124
Tomatoes						
Tomatoes (1 lb.)	91	19.4	0.8	0	0	12
Boiled, without salt (1 cup)	63	13.3	0.5	0	0	10
Canned, low sodium, *Featherweight* (½ cup)	20	4.0	0	0	0	10
Paste, canned, *Contadina* (6 oz.)	150	35.0	0	0	0	69
Paste, canned, *Del Monte* (6 oz.)	150	34.0	1.0	NA	0	25
Paste, canned, *Featherweight* (6 oz.)	150	35.0	0	0	0	68
● Pear, canned, *Contadina* (8 oz.)	50	11.0	0	0	0	358
Pieces, frozen, low-sodium, *Winter Garden Pipe n' Ready* (3.2 oz.)	20	4.0	0	0	0	5
● Puree, canned (16 oz.)	177	40.4	0.9	0	0	1809
Puree, canned, *Featherweight* (1 cup)	90	20.0	0	0	0	10
Puree, canned, low-sodium (16 oz.)	177	40.4	0.9	0	0	27
Puree, heavy, canned, *Contadina* (8 oz.)	100	24.0	0	0	0	43
●★Sauce, canned, *Contadina* (4 oz.)	40	9.0	0	0	0	500
●★Stewed, canned, *Del Monte* (1 cup)	70	16.0	0	0	0	765

Alerts: ● Sodium ★ Sugar ■ Cholesterol

Food Description	Calories	Carbohydrates (grams)	Fat (grams)	Saturated Fat (grams)	Cholesterol (milligrams)	Sodium (milligrams)
●★Stewed, canned, *Stokely-Van Camp* (1 cup)	70	15.0	0	0	0	440
●★Wedges, canned, juice pack, *Del Monte* (1 cup)	60	14.0	0	0	0	475
Whole, canned, low sodium, *Nutradiet* (½ cup)	25	5.0	0	0	0	15
●Whole, canned, *Stokely-Van Camp* (1 cup)	50	10.0	0	0	0	380
Turnip greens (1 lb.)	127	22.7	1.4	0	0	322
Turnip greens, boiled briefly, without salt, drained (1 cup)	29	5.2	0.3	0	0	72
●Turnip greens, chopped, canned, *Stokely-Van Camp* (1 cup)	35	6.0	1.0	NA	0	650
Turnip greens, chopped, frozen, *Birds Eye* (3.3 oz.)	20	3.0	0	0	0	10
Turnip greens, leaf, cut, frozen, *Winter Garden* (3.3 oz.)	20	3.0	0	0	0	11
Turnips, boiled, without salt, drained, mashed (1 cup)	53	11.3	0.5	0	0	78
Turnips, chopped, frozen, *Winter Garden* (3.2 oz.)	20	3.0	0	0	0	14
Turnips, cubed, boiled, without salt, drained (1 cup)	36	7.6	0.3	0	0	52
Waterchestnuts, Chinese (1 lb.)	276	66.4	0.7	0	0	69
Watercress, leaves and stems (1 cup)	7	1.0	0.1	0	0	18
Wax Beans						
Boiled, without salt, drained (1 cup)	28	5.8	0.3	0	0	4
Cut, frozen, *Birds Eye* (3 oz.)	30	4.0	0	0	0	2
●French cut, canned, *Del Monte* (1 cup)	35	7.0	0	0	0	665
Frozen (9 oz.)	35	8.1	0.1	0	0	1
Pieces, canned, low sodium, *Featherweight* (½ cup)	25	5.0	0	0	0	10
●Sliced, canned, *Stokely-Van Camp* (1 cup)	35	7.0	0	0	0	845
Winter squash, baked, without salt, mashed (1 cup)	129	31.6	0.8	0	0	2
Winter squash, boiled, without salt, mashed (1 cup)	93	22.5	0.7	0	0	2

Alerts: ● Sodium ★ Sugar ■ Cholesterol

Food Description	Calories	Carbohydrates (grams)	Fat (grams)	Saturated Fat (grams)	Cholesterol (milligrams)	Sodium (milligrams)
Winter squash, frozen (12 oz. package)	129	31.3	1.0	0	0	3
Yams						
★In heavy syrup, canned, *Royal Prince, Joan of Arc* (½ cup)	147	35.0	0	0	0	57
★In orange/pineapple sauce, canned, *Royal Prince, Joan of Arc* (½ cup)	180	44.0	0	0	0	30
★In syrup, canned, *Sugary Sam* (1 cup)	210	55.0	1.0	NA	0	NA
★Sliced, frozen, *Winter Garden* (3.2 oz.)	90	21.0	0	0	0	6
Zucchini, frozen, *Birds Eye 5 Minute* (3.3 oz.)	16	3.0	0	0	0	2
●★Zucchini, sliced, canned, *Del Monte* (1 cup)	60	16.0	0	0	0	850
Zucchini, sliced, frozen, *Winter Garden* (3.3 oz.)	16	3.0	0	0	0	2
Zucchini squash, sliced (1 cup)	22	4.7	0.1	0	0	1
VEGETABLE DISHES AND COMBINATIONS						
●★■Asparagus souffle, frozen, *Stouffers* (4 oz.)	115	8.0	7.0	NA	NA	440
Broccoli and cauliflower, frozen, *Winter Garden* (3.2 oz.)	25	4.0	0	0	0	19
●★Broccoli and cheese, frozen, *Mrs. Paul's Light Batter* (2.5 oz.)	150	18.0	7.0	NA	NA	575
●★Broccoli, au gratin, frozen, *Stouffers* (5 oz.)	170	9.0	12.0	NA	NA	470
●★Broccoli, with cheese sauce, frozen, *Birds Eye* (3.3 oz.)	110	8.0	8.0	NA	NA	440
●★Cantonese style, stir-fry, with seasonings, frozen, *Birds Eye* (3.3 oz.)	50	11.0	0	0	0	470
●★Carrots, with brown sugar glaze, frozen, *Birds Eye* (3.3 oz.)	80	15.0	2.0	NA	NA	500
●★Cauliflower, au gratin, frozen, *Stouffers* (5 oz.)	155	11.0	10.0	NA	NA	445
●★Cauliflower, with cheese sauce, frozen, *Birds Eye* (3.3 oz.)	110	9.0	7.0	NA	NA	420

Alerts: ● Sodium ★ Sugar ■ Cholesterol

Food Description	Calories	Carbohydrates (grams)	Fat (grams)	Saturated Fat (grams)	Cholesterol (milligrams)	Sodium (milligrams)
●★ Cauliflower, with cheese sauce, frozen, *Green Giant* (3½ oz.)	52	5.6	2.3	NA	NA	324
● Chinese, frozen, *La Choy* (10 oz.)	72	10.5	0.8	0	NA	1552
● Chinese style, stir-fry, frozen, *Birds Eye* (3.3 oz.)	30	7.0	0	0	NA	500
●★ Corn and peppers, canned, *Del Monte* (1 cup)	190	40.0	1.0	NA	0	435
●★ Corn and sweet peppers, canned, *Mexicorn, Green Giant* (3½ oz.)	86	17.9	0.5	0	0	309
●★ Corn jubilee, frozen, *Birds Eye* (3.3 oz.)	120	16.0	5.0	NA	NA	280
●★■ Corn souffle, frozen, *Stouffers* (4 oz.)	155	19.0	7.0	NA	NA	510
●★ Danish style, with seasoned sauce, frozen, *Birds Eye* (3.3 oz.)	45	9.0	0	0	NA	320
●★■ Eggplant parmesan, frozen, *Mrs. Paul's* (5½ oz.)	250	21.0	16.0	NA	NA	1100
● French cut green beans and almonds, with seasonings, frozen, *Birds Eye* (3 oz.)	50	8.0	2.0	NA	NA	335
● Green beans and mushrooms, casserole, frozen, *Stouffers* (4¾ oz.)	150	12.0	9.0	NA	NA	675
Green beans and new potatoes, frozen, *Winter Garden* (3.2 oz.)	40	9.0	0	0	0	5
● Green peas and mushrooms, with seasonings, frozen, *Birds Eye* (3.3 oz.)	70	13.0	0	0	NA	240
●★ Green pepper, stuffed with beef, frozen, *Green Giant* (3½ oz.)	101	9.1	5.4	NA	NA	462
●★ Italian style, with sauce, frozen, *Birds Eye International Recipes* (3.3 oz.)	60	9.0	1.0	NA	NA	475
●★ Japanese, frozen, *La Choy* (10 oz.)	72	11.6	0.3	NA	NA	1224
★ Japanese, frozen, *Stokely-Van Camp* (3.2 oz.)	25	5.0	0	0	0	34
●★ Japanese style, stir-fry, frozen, *Birds Eye* (3.3 oz.)	30	6.0	0	0	NA	515

Alerts: ● Sodium ★ Sugar ■ Cholesterol

Food Description	Calories	Carbohydrates (grams)	Fat (grams)	Saturated Fat (grams)	Cholesterol (milligrams)	Sodium (milligrams)
★*Milano,* frozen, *Stokely-Van Camp* (3.2 oz.)	45	9.0	0	0	0	32
Mixed Vegetables						
●★Canned, *Del Monte* (1 cup)	80	16.0	1.0	NA	0	625
★Canned, low sodium, *Featherweight* (½ cup)	40	8.0	0	0	0	25
●★Canned, *Stokely-Van Camp* (1 cup)	80	17.0	0	0	0	245
★Frozen, *Birds Eye* (3.3 oz.)	60	11.0	0	0	0	45
★Frozen, *Stokely-Van Camp* (3.3 oz.)	60	12.0	0	0	0	50
★Frozen, *Winter Garden* (3.3 oz.)	60	13.0	0	0	0	52
●★With butter sauce, frozen, *Green Giant* (3½ oz.)	65	9.0	2.2	NA	NA	352
●★With onion sauce, frozen, *Birds Eye* (2.6 oz.)	110	13.0	5.0	NA	NA	340
●★New England style, *Birds Eye American Recipe* (3.3 oz.)	70	12.0	1.0	NA	NA	320
Okra and tomatoes, frozen, *Winter Garden* (3.2 oz.)	25	5.0	0	0	0	6
●★Okra gumbo, frozen, *Green Giant Southern Recipe* (3½ oz.)	90	5.6	7.0	NA	NA	356
●★Onions, small, with cream sauce, frozen, *Birds Eye* (3 oz.)	100	11.0	6.0	NA	NA	335
★*Parisian,* frozen, *Stokely-Van Camp* (3.2 oz.)	30	6.0	0	0	0	24
●★Peas and carrots, canned, *Del Monte* (1 cup)	100	19.0	0	0	0	630
★Peas and carrots, canned, low sodium, *Nutradiet* (½ cup)	35	7.0	0	0	0	10
●★Peas and carrots, frozen, *Birds Eye* (3.3 oz.)	50	9.0	0	0	0	90
★Peas and cauliflower, frozen, *Winter Garden* (3.2 oz.)	60	9.0	0	0	0	44
★Peas, creme, frozen, *Winter Garden* (3.3 oz.)	130	23.0	1.0	NA	NA	6
●★Peas, green, with cream sauce, frozen, *Birds Eye* (2.6 oz.)	130	14.0	7.0	NA	NA	420
Potatoes						
●★Au gratin, *Big Tate* (⅙ package)	110	18.0	3.0	NA	NA	500

Alerts: ● Sodium ★ Sugar ■ Cholesterol

Food Description	Calories	Carbohydrates (grams)	Fat (grams)	Saturated Fat (grams)	Cholesterol (milligrams)	Sodium (milligrams)
●★Au gratin, frozen, *Stouffers* (3¾ oz.)	135	13.0	8.0	NA	NA	480
●★Au gratin, mix, prepared, *Betty Crocker* (½ cup)	150	21.0	6.0	NA	NA	605
●★Hash brown, mix, *Big Tate* (⅙ package)	100	22.0	0	0	NA	435
●★Hash brown, mix, prepared, *Betty Crocker* (½ cup)	150	22.0	6.0	NA	NA	455
Mashed, Idaho, *French's* (mix for ½ cup)	60	15.0	0	0	NA	30
● Mashed, prepared, *Betty Crocker Potato Buds* (½ cup)	130	15.0	6.0	NA	NA	355
● Mashed, prepared, *Hungry Jack* (½ cup)	140	16.0	7.0	NA	NA	375
●★Scalloped, *Big Tate* (⅙ package)	100	21.0	0	0	NA	440
●★Scalloped, dehydrated, *Betty Crocker* (⅙ package)	90	18.0	1.0	NA	NA	520
●★Scalloped, frozen, *Stouffers* (4 oz.)	126	14.0	7.0	NA	NA	450
●★Stuffed with chives and sour cream, frozen, *Green Giant Bake 'N Serve* (3½ oz.)	164	21.1	7.4	NA	NA	390
●★*Romano*, frozen, *Stokely-Van Camp* (3.2 oz.)	40	9.0	0	0	0	70
●★San Francisco style, *Birds Eye American Recipe* (3.3 oz.)	50	8.0	1.0	NA	NA	305
●★Spinach, creamed, frozen, *Green Giant* (3½ oz.)	74	8.3	3.2	NA	NA	400
●★■Spinach souffle, frozen, *Stouffers* (4 oz.)	135	12.0	7.0	NA	NA	600
★Succotash, frozen, *Birds Eye 5 Minute* (3.3 oz.)	80	17.0	1.0	NA	NA	25
★Succotash, frozen, *Stokely-Van Camp* (3.3 oz.)	100	21.0	0	0	0	45
●★Sweet peas and sliced carrots, canned, *Freshlike* (1 cup)	80	19.0	0	NA	NA	NA
●★Sweet peas and sliced carrots, canned, *Veg-All* (1 cup)	80	19.0	0	NA	NA	NA

Alerts: ● Sodium   ★ Sugar   ■ Cholesterol